WITH CHILD: BIRTH THROUGH THE AGES

WITH CHILD

BIRTH THROUGH THE AGES

JENNY CARTER and THÉRÈSE DURIEZ

MAINSTREAM PUBLISHING

First published in 1986 by
MAINSTREAM PUBLISHING COMPANY
(EDINBURGH) LTD.
7 Albany Street
Edinburgh EH1 3UG

Carter, Jenny
  With child, birth through the ages.
  1. Childbirth—History
  I. Title   II. Duriez, Thérése
  618.4'09   RG651

  ISBN 0-906391-90-3

Typeset in 11/12 Garamond by Mainstream Publishing.
Printed by Billing & Sons, Ltd. Worcester.

CONTENTS

Picture acknowledgements

The author and publishers would like to thank the following for permission to reproduce material on the pages indicated: BBC Hulton Picture Library, back cover, 79, 113, 115, 121, 126, 127, 129, 130, 131, 145, 159, 160, 164, 165, 213, 216; Bibliotheque Forney, 13; British Museum, courtesy of the Trustees, 199, 203, 207, 208; Professor Ian Donald, 192; Centre for Reproductive Biology, 189; David Brock and Roger Sutcliffe, 191, Durex Contraception Information Service, 220-1, Frederique Leboyer, 180; Greater London Council photograph Library, 150; Sally and Richard Greenhill Photo Library, 193; The Labour Party, 157; Professor Hugh McLaren, 235; Mansell Collection, 19, 37, 39, 40, 81, 93, 95, 96, 98, 99, 111, 117, 119, 120, 123, 125; The Medical Archives Office, University of Glasgow, 34, 143, 151, 175, 251; Michel Odent, 182; Radcliffe College, Cambridge, Massachusetts, 168; Royal Society of Medicine, 147; Dora Rusell, 233; Patrick Steptoe and Professor Robert Edwards, 239, 241.

For the men in our lives
Mike, Christopher, Plum and Roy.

INTRODUCTION

A WOMAN approaching motherhood today is faced with a wealth of
literature on the subject: every few months, another birth manual will
appear on the shelves, propounding some new philosophy, explaining,
educating, instructing — and the sheer volume of it all can be as
confusing as it is helpful.

As mothers ourselves — and mothers who had to have recourse to
modern technology for the safety of our babies — we felt that the 'nature
is all' philosophy of birth was in some respects lacking. Why, after
centuries of 'natural birth', do women want to return to it? What was
childbirth really like for women in the past? How do the modern
'methods' fit into the huge span of history, into all the long years before
modern birth technology, hospital deliveries and Caesarean section,
before obstetrician and episiotomy?

Today most women in the western world have a baby when they
choose to. A woman may choose to have her baby in her home, as women
have for centuries, or she may deliver the baby in hospital. She may
choose to give birth standing up, lying down, or even under water. She
may choose to have a midwife present or a doctor, her husband or her
entire family. Women have never had so much freedom of choice where
childbirth is concerned.

Of course, women may still be as apprehensive as they are excited
about their baby's arrival: but no-one today expects to die. Yet as little as
seventy years ago, a woman facing birth knew that she might also be
facing death. 'I always prepared myself to die, and I think this awful
depression is common to most at this time,' said one mother in 1914.
(WCG, *Maternity: Letters from Working Women,* London 1978, p166).
After all, when birth was straightforward, all was well. If anything began
to go wrong, though, what could be done?

The local midwife might be sent scurrying off for ergot to speed the
contractions, or she might just try to pull on the part of the baby which
presented itself most conveniently. Pushed to extremes, she might
abandon the woman to her fate — or, almost equally horrific, she would

send for the nearest barber-surgeon with his knives and hooks. Even if the mother had a 'normal' delivery, she was still open to the dangers of death from infection or haemorrhage. After all, there were no antibiotics or blood transfusions available until a mere fifty years ago.

The development of medical knowledge has played a key part in the modern western woman's attitude to and expectations of birth. Now she can reasonably rely on expert technology in surgical techniques, pain-killing drugs, basic hygiene, prenatal diagnosis and a thorough understanding of her body and how it works. Yet few of the facilities we now take for granted were available to women even as recently as the beginning of this century.

There are many who will argue, of course, that in the search for the 'ideal' pain-free birth, too much has been sacrificed, and that the male-dominated world of medicine has taken over what is essentially woman's business. We are now witnessing a struggle for power in the place and process of birth.

For centuries it *was* women who controlled birth. Few men were involved in labour and delivery until medical knowledge began to make significant advances in the mid-nineteenth century. Where the midwife had once been in charge, now she began to find herself struggling for her very existence. Doctors, meanwhile, in command of the new emerging technology, consolidated their control. Women believed that hospitals held the key to safe, pain-free delivery. The emerging specialists — obstetricians — encouraged women to turn increasingly to hospitals for the delivery of their children. Birth became a clinical event, and in some places hospital routines were imposed which institutionalised and dehumanised the birth process. Anaesthetics, while they removed pain, also removed the experience of delivery altogether. And so finally women, with their new high expectations of safety, began to demand a better birth experience.

Accompanying medical advance have been improvements in social conditions. A concern for diet and decent living conditions, improvements in housing, in sanitation and in general welfare have made women stronger, more able to cope with the rigours of childbearing. In addition, the ability to exert a degree of control over their own fertility — through contraception, sterilisation or, if needs must, abortion — has reduced the drastically debilitating effects of multiparity (bearing many children).

The last few decades have seen the publication of a considerable amount of material on the issues which affect childbirth — medical, social, political. Many are highly specialised documents, appearing in the pages of professional journals; others are impressive pieces of research by men and women in the academic world. What, it seemed to us, was lacking was a book which presented an overall picture of these changes, a book which was simple enough for everyone to understand, and was easy to assimilate.

Modern medicine evolved from the work of the ancient Egyptians and Greeks, which provided medical researchers in Europe with the foundations of their new science. It was in Europe that the major developments in modern medicine took place. For centuries childbirth remained outwith the province of medicine, but by the seventeenth century medical enquiry was beginning to turn to the birth process.

The early chapters of *With Child* set the scene for the revolution in birth technology which took place in western industrial society in the twentieth century. The experiences of women in western European pre-industrial society form the early chapters of the book, with particular emphasis on the seventeenth and eighteenth centuries. Until that period birth practices had changed little. In the course of researching the book, certain themes began to emerge; in particular, the gradual erosion of the position of the midwife as birth technology became more complex. The role of the midwife is still viewed as fundamental, and the reasons for her diminishing responsibility merited a separate section. Similarly, the increasing complexity of medical knowledge had a direct bearing on the birth process — infection, anaesthesia, surgery — and also required to be dealt with in some detail.

The amount of material available for a book of this nature is vast; as modern methods evolved, it became increasingly impossible to deal in detail with changes in not only medicine but society, economics and politics in every European country. In Britain, changes in medicine ran parallel to social upheaval caused by the Industrial Revolution and, in the twentieth century, to the advent of the Welfare State and the National Health Service which had a fundamental effect on health in general and lives of women in particular. In America, which emerged as a nation only in the late eighteenth century, the assumption of control of the birth process by men is of particular interest. We have chosen, therefore, to look in the twentieth century, primarily at what happened in Britain and America, while taking account of the very important contributions of France and other countries.

The final section of the book, 'Fertility and Choice' deals with abortion, birth control and infertility. An examination of fertility is inseparable from pregnancy and the birth process. The effects of constant childbearing on women in past centuries was totally debilitating, and the possibility of choice is critically important to the improvement of women's health generally and their performance in birth in particular.

Birth processes in eastern and third world countries developed along lines very different to those in western society. To deal with a large range of cultural practices was not possible in a book of this extent. But it is interesting to note that changes in western society are already having a profound effect on these cultures. Women we have spoken to from Africa, Sudan, Oman, China and elsewhere have told us that the ancient traditions of home birth are already being abandoned in favour of the hospital.

With Child draws together the strands from many centuries of history, showing how dramatic the change in birth has been, and giving a perspective to the issues we all face today.

In our research, we have been greatly indebted to many friends and colleagues for their help and encouragement. In particular we would like to thank Sir Dugald Baird for allowing us to interview him; Mr Frank Loeffler, Consultant Obstetrician and Gynaecologist at St Mary's, Paddington, and Queen Charlotte's Hospital, London; Dr Martin Lees, Consultant Obstetrician and Gynaecologist at Simpson Memorial Maternity Hospital, Edinburgh; Dr Derek Dow at the Medical Archives Office, University of Glasgow; Dr Ian Stevenson, Senior Lecturer, General Practice Unit, University of Edinburgh; Dr Judy Bury, Counsellor, Brook Advisory Services, Edinburgh; Mrs Maisie Haley, District Nursing Officer, Perthshire. We are also extremely grateful for advice and guidance from the History Department and the History of Medicine Department at the University of Edinburgh, and the Social Sciences Department at Napier College, Edinburgh. We would like to thank Basic Books, Inc, New York for allowing us to use material from *A History of Women's Bodies* by Edward Shorter and The Free Press, New York for allowing us to use material from *Lying-in: A History of childbirth in America* by Richard W Wertz and Dorothy C Wertz. To Robert Thomson we would like to give our thanks for allowing us to quote parts of his mother's unpublished manuscript, *Stork's Nest.* And in particular we wish to acknowledge the patience and fortitude of our families during the long months spent working on the book.

EVE'S LEGACY

Adam was not deceived, but the woman was deceived and became a transgressor. Yet woman will be saved through bearing children, if she continues in faith and love and holiness, with modesty.

Holy Bible, 1 Timothy 2, 14-18.

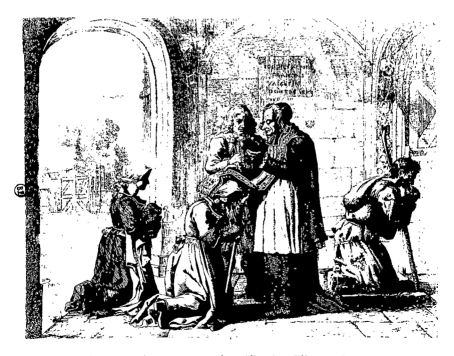

A woman undergoing the ceremony of purification. The mother remained at the door of the church until the priest or pastor fetched her and brought her to the altar. (Engraving by Oliver Perrin, 'Galerie bretonne', 1808)

WOMEN IN SOCIETY

'Sin came through a woman, but salvation through a virgin.'[1]

Throughout history a woman's most important function has been the bearing of children. Today the majority of women in western society have the ability to choose when to have their children: in the past, lacking any real control over their own fertility, childbearing was a constant and debilitating process. Nor was it one that seems to have won her much respect — on the contrary, over the centuries, it became her only justification.

The idea that woman is inferior to man has a long history — the Ancient Greeks, for example, regarded women as physically, intellectually and morally weaker than men — but the adoption of Christianity by western society introduced a new argument in favour of the subjugation of women with its interpretations of the Fall and the guilt of Eve. Because Eve had introduced sin into the world it was the role of women to atone for her sin, in particular in childbirth. The development of moral attitudes to women bolstered by Genesis and the narrative of the temptation, together with certain statements in the writings of St Paul, must be held largely responsible for the burden of guilt with which women were saddled.[2]

The early Church emerged as a force as the civilisation of Rome declined and the barbarian tribes of Europe and North Asia began four hundred years of strife. In these so-called 'Dark Ages', Christian values became a useful means of imposing order on a society in chaos. Gradually the Church, after the fall of Rome in the 5th century AD, became organised into an ecclesiastical hierarchy patterned on the structure of the Roman empire. Any divergence from the Church's teaching was seen as a real threat to the stability of society. A number of heresies encouraged women to preach, baptise and prophesy and as these were suppressed women were actively discouraged from any active involvement in the Church.

The wave of asceticism that swept over the early Church was an important influence on attitudes towards women. Christian theologians such as Jerome, Ambrose and Augustine in the fourth century inherited this strong ascetic tradition coupled with a fear of the temptations woman offered. Dedicating their lives to chastity, they saw little in the lifestyles of Roman women to temper their disparagement of them. Jerome was unwaveringly severe on womankind: 'One man among a thousand I found, but one woman among all these I have not found.'[3]

So great was the ascetic ideal and fear of woman as the temptress that matrimony could not wholly surmount it. Virginity became the ideal; and in the fourth and fifth centuries a new cult developed which exalted Mary, the new Eve, a virgin protected throughout life from every physical or spiritual contamination. Mary was the model of behaviour, an ideal unattainable to any other women — yet veneration for her did not change or improve the way in which women in general were regarded.

Well into the Middle Ages women were recommended to turn away from marriage as the lesser good. The author of *Hali Meidenhaad* (Holy Maidenhood), a thirteenth-century English treatise on virginity, drew attention to the fleshly burden of bearing and rearing children:

> Thy ruddy face shall turn lean, and grow green as grass.
> Thine eyes shall be dusky and underneath grow pale;
> And by the giddiness of thy brain thy head shall ache sorely.[4]

Labour was presented as a frightening or painful ordeal when a woman was subjected to the 'indelicate skill' of the midwife.

The Church's fear of woman's sexuality was particularly evident in its attitude to menstruation and childbirth. There were many ancient taboos on women: Hebrew law forbade couples to have intercourse when a woman was menstruating and the Greeks and Romans regarded menstruation as a blight. Because of its fears of contamination by woman's demonic powers, the early Church invoked rules to keep women away from sacred objects while menstruating and they were only allowed to receive communion through a veil. Centuries later mediaeval writers described the monsters that would be born to those who had intercourse during menstruation, and the way in which such children would suffer from leprosy or epilepsy.

Instead of embracing a woman in childbirth, the Church reiterated Hebrew Law which had stipulated that a woman could not enter a church for thirty-three days after giving birth to a son, or sixty-six days after the birth of a daughter. As a woman neared delivery she was advised to take communion. Death was always a possibility, and from the moment labour began a woman was in an unclean state spiritually. So in addition to her physical trauma a woman experienced the spiritual trauma of being excluded from the Christian community.

Nor did the Church display much interest in the mother during birth. By the Middle Ages the main concern was to have the baby baptised, and when it was a choice between the life of the mother and the child, midwives were advised to save the baby. In 1280 the Council of Boulogne decreed that when a mother died in childbirth, her mouth should be held open so that the baby would not suffocate while a Caesarean was attempted.

Women who died in childbirth or even during pregnancy were often denied burial in consecrated ground, or were buried in a part of the graveyard reserved for murderers and suicides. Because such women were unclean there was a fear of the emanations that could come from their bodies. Humane Churchmen urged acceptance of corpses but often without success. In parts of Europe such practices continued until the eighteenth century.

After giving birth a woman still had to wait six to eight weeks for the ceremony of purification before she was allowed to re-enter the body of the Church.

Those women who did not dedicate their lives to religion and chastity were placed in a cleft stick. Marriage was debased but the bearing of children was the most important justification for marriage and also offered the best means of escaping from the weight of original sin. On the other hand, bearing children entailed spiritual risks because during birth a woman was not in a state of grace. There were also numerous restrictions on when intercourse was permissable. It has been worked out that by the fourteenth century coition was allowed by the Church on only 200 days per year, not taking into account voluntary abstentions.

From the middle of the thirteenth century there had been attempts made within the Church to raise marriage from its lowly position. It began to be seen as a desirable condition worthy of blessing. Mary was portrayed not only as a virgin mother but as the model for the excellence of the married state. Certainly, payment of the marriage debt had always been given some recognition. Even St Paul had said:

> The husband should give to the wife her conjugal rights, and likewise the wife to her husband. For the wife does not rule over her own body but the husband does. Likewise the husband does not rule over his own body, but the wife does.[5]

The Canterbury Tales, written in the fourteenth century, shows the continuing concern of society in such matters. Chaucer's parson says that his wife:

> ... has the merit of chastity who yields the debt of the body to her husband, yes, though it be contrary to her liking and the desire of her heart.[6]

Indeed his Wife of Bath is very determined that she should receive what is her right:

> In wifehood I intend to use my instrument as generously as my maker sent it. If I am niggardly, may God give me sorrow! My husband shall have it morning and night when it pleases him to come forth and pay his debt.[7]

The Wife of Bath's practicality in matters of sex, however, is coupled with her desire to dominate her husband, and she is portrayed as a compendium of all women's vices.

Although the concept of romantic love began to gain ground in the twelfth century in accompaniment with the ideal of knighthood, lay literature had a long legacy of misogyny inherited from classical times.

Mediaeval preachers and theologians took this up and as a consequence they 'presented a picture of womanhood, ill-balanced indeed, but sufficiently realistic and lively to appeal to the lay mind.'[8]

It has been argued that much of the misogyny of mediaeval literature was part of a 'courtly game': women were condemned 'not because there is anything intrinsically evil about women but because women may easily be regarded as a source of fleshly rather than spiritual satisfaction.'[9] However, any real assessment of women's lives and how much they were affected by the views propounded by theologians is difficult because of their exclusion from public life and the lack of records of the lives of the mass of women.

Many of the treatises on virginity argued that it would allow freedom not only for a life of spirituality but also from the dominance of a husband. The number of women who, during the 'Dark Ages', responded to the call is probably an indication that they valued their independence. Certainly it was the convents rather than secular life which produced so many prominent and powerful women in the Middle Ages.

In secular life there are instances of women who wielded power. Even allowing that these were exceptions, men cannot have placed women in as little regard as much writing might suggest. Social position is more influenced by the pressures of everyday life than theoretical views. Among the poor a rough equality was needed to make a meagre living from the land, and middle-class women often ran households and businesses single-handed when their menfolk were away, assuming considerable responsibility. Whatever the attitude taken by the Church, female evangelism also revived, and there were women preachers. Many Churchmen, too, were not opposed to the idea of conjugal love; and that notion became increasingly evident in the vernacular literature.

Yet the belief that women were innately inferior did not lose its appeal. During the thirteenth century it was fuelled by translations of Aristotle's *Historia Animalium* in which the female of the species was described as a 'misbegotten male', a biological imperfection. The male seed ordinarily bred other males, other perfect beings, but if the sperm was flawed or affected by accident or climate, a female was formed instead. The female was merely a host nursing the child in her womb until the time of birth: the real parent was considered to be the father. Married women could not inherit or pass on property: they were non-existent in the face of the law. They were subject to their husbands and fathers and could be beaten for any number of reasons: failing to comply with matrimonial plans, not conforming to their husband's ideas about behaviour, and even for giving birth to a mentally handicapped child.[10] Moverover, women accepted their position in the natural hierarchy — below the angels and man but above the animals — because of the circumstances of Eve's creation and sin.

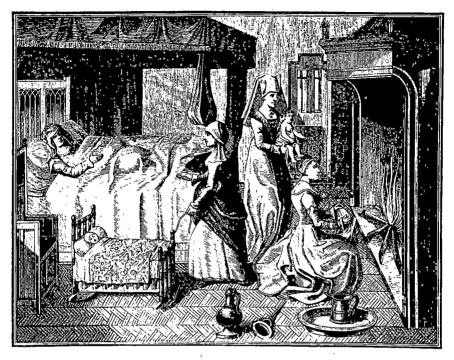

A typical birth scene with the new mother and baby being attended by women.
For centuries birthing was conducted exclusively by women. (From a miniature
of Histoire de la Belle Helene, *a fifteenth century manuscript.)*

The belief that the whole end of sex was procreation did not diminish
over the centuries. If anything, it was increased from the sixteenth
century by the Puritan emphasis on the biblical injunction to increase and
multiply their followers. The desire for children within marriage, as
many and as quickly as possible, was common throughout society.

In fact because childbearing was regarded as the way in which women
found redemption, infertility was often equated with lack of grace.
Manuals and almanacs filled with remedies for the childless abounded.
Despite the burden constant pregnancy placed on women, it was the
childless woman who was felt to be disadvantaged.

WHAT WAS BIRTH LIKE?

> In the past women gave birth to their children at home. There
> among family and friends, they were not 'patients' and childbirth
> was not an 'illness'. It was a natural process.[1]

The religious emphasis given to procreation and the lack of reliable birth control ensured that the lives of most women in the past were dominated by a cycle of pregnancy and birth. 'Childbirth was part of the natural order of things',[2] but over the centuries the process became imbued with traditional beliefs inherited from the Greeks and Romans and steeped in superstitions and the practice of magic. It has been suggested that these practices restricted the control a mother had over her own delivery and that far from being left to the care of nature a mother was often

> harassed by meddlers and officious interveners from the moment she was pregnant until she finally received her ritual cleansing a month after giving birth.[3]

Pregnancy

For the majority of women, pregnancy before the twentieth century afforded little chance of special treatment and antenatal care was virtually non-existent.

About the only practice common throughout the social spectrum, was bleeding. This entailed opening a vein with a knife and drawing off a pint or two of blood because it was believed that illness was caused by a plethora of blood. In some areas bleeding was used until well into the nineteenth century. It was used to treat symptoms like headaches, palpitation, singing in the ears and shortness of breath. The frequency of bleeding varied, but because it had become so much a part of traditional practice most women wanted to be bled at least once and often as many as seven or eight times during a pregnancy. Even when there were no symptoms to treat, women would demand it because of the popular belief that otherwise the child would drown in an excess of blood during delivery.[4]

During the eighteenth century some writers began to give advice to pregnant women on health care. In 1747 Dr William Cadogan, an English doctor, recommended the virtues of fresh vegetables and fruit, clean linen and fresh air, and in his *Treatise on Midwifery*, published in 1781, Alexander Hamilton, Professor of Midwifery at Edinburgh, gave advice which holds good today:

> Women when pregnant should lead a regular and temperate life carefully avoiding whatever is to disagree with the stomach; they should breathe a free open air; their company should be agreeable and cheerful; their exercise should be moderate, and adapted to their particular situation; they should, especially in the early months when the connection between ovum and womb is feeble, avoid crowds, confinement, every situation which renders them under any disagreeable restriction; agitation of body from violent or improper exercise . . . and whatever disturbs either the body or mind.

In later pregnancy, Hamilton went on, women should,

> When heavy or unwieldy, troubled with pains, cramps or swelled
> legs, (have) frequent rest on a bed or couch through the day; and in
> the night, the posture of the body should be frequently changed, that
> the womb may be prevented from constantly pressing on any part.[5]

Such counselling can have benefited only a minority of women. Economic restraints did not allow most women to rest during pregnancy. Particularly in country areas, women would often work till labour began: 'You often see women just a few days before their delivery sweating in the fields or stumbling homeward under some heavy load of fodder.'[6] In fact many women worked hardest towards the end of pregnancy because it was commonly believed that intense physical labour made for an easier birth.

Similarly, it took centuries for advice about diet to take effect although in some areas it was customary to indulge a pregnant woman's cravings. In parts of Germany, for instance, it was stipulated in law that a pregnant woman had certain food rights. She was allowed to pick fruit when she wanted, and her husband was allowed to violate the hunting and fishing laws to provide extra food. A better-off woman might be given delicacies such as pork or vegetable stew, eggs and fruit.[7]

However, particularly in the seventeenth and early eighteenth centuries, the diet of both women and men in country areas was held in a precarious balance following a downturn in the economy which began at the end of the Middle Ages. Developments in food production did lead to an improvement in diet during the eighteenth century. The potato and other root crops were introduced as was rye bread. Together with the salted pork put away at the annual slaughter these items added variety to the diet and starvation became a rarity.

Yet even after a minimally adequate diet became available, it has been suggested that women did less well than men.[8] The man was the bread-winner and the master of the house in pre-industrial Europe. It was customary to give him the lion's share of the food, particularly food of a high nutrient value. At mealtimes women were usually served last and often received not only the worst but least. In consequence women were often undernourished and less able than men to resist infection and maintain an adequate level of physical energy. Even pregnant women received little consideration. In some areas it was recorded that women had to survive on a diet of 'legumes, weak bread dishes and water or bad beer'[9] and that sometimes their diet was 'scarcely better than that of the livestock'.[10] Lack of proper nutrition meant that some mothers were unable to ensure their babies reached the necessary body weight at birth and many babies died before or soon after birth for this reason.

In addition to the lack of care and attention, a pregnant woman often had to contend with the web of superstitious beliefs which were guaranteed to fill her with fears and misgivings.

In country areas particularly, the belief that a woman's emotions or environment could harm her unborn child physically or spiritually imposed numerous constraints. For example, if she was startled by a dog jumping her baby would have 'dog feet'; if she looked at the moon she would give birth to a lunatic or sleepwalker,[11] and if she became a godmother to another woman's baby one of the babies, born or unborn, would die.[12]

Birth

The majority of women, whatever their social status, gave birth in the home until the twentieth century. In the larger, wealthier houses of Europe birth usually took place in the main bedroom and the midwife might come to stay some time before the birth. The woman's mother and relations would also come to be 'her comforter and overseer in her great extremity'.[13] Similarly, in seventeenth-century colonial America friends and relations often travelled some distance to help the mother and take over her household duties. Birth there normally took place in the borning room, a small room behind the central chimney which was partitioned off from the living areas to keep it free from draughts. In peasant societies women seldom had the opportunity for such preparations but when the birth began friends and relations would gather round and sometimes as many as thirty people were present. In these homes there was rarely a choice of rooms and birth often took place on the bare floor, or on sacks of hay.

Once the labour began the main feature of the birthing chamber was the insistence on heat.

> When the woman is in labour, she is often attended by a number of her friends in a small room, with a large fire which, together with her own pains, throw her into profuse sweats; by the heat of the chamber, and the breath of so many people, the whole air is rendered foul and unfit for respiration . . .[14]

Any hint of fresh air was traditionally regarded with terror. Writing in 1784 Bernard Faust, a male midwife, commented:

> How marvellous it is when mothers leave the windows of their bedrooms open. Then the stand-offish old women, who otherwise crowd round the mother in a room they have heated to boiling point, will now stay home, for they dread these cool rooms, cleansed with fresh air, more fearfully than if one were burning asafetida.[15]

There are records well into the twentieth century which show that the fire had pride of place in the birthing room.

Disregarding the old women who often increased the mother's fear with tales of obstetric disaster, the duty of the attendants was to minister to the mother and help her as best they could. The mother might be walked round the room, have her back massaged or be given special food and cordials.

According to one of the earliest birth manuals, *The Byrth of Mankynde* published in 1545, the principal attendant, the midwife, should:

> sit before the labouring woman and shall diligently observe and wait,
> how much and after what means the child stireth itself. Also shall
> with hands anoynted with the oyle of those white lillies, rule and
> direct everything as shall seme best. Also the midwife must instruct
> and comfort the party not only refreshing her with good meat and
> drink, but also with sweet words giving her hope of a good speedie
> deliverance, encouraging and enstomacking her to patience and
> tolerance, bidding her to hold her breath as much as she may, also
> stroking gently with her hands her belly about the navel for that
> helps to depress the birth downward.[16]

She might also apply warm cloths to the stomach or administer an enema to widen the birth canal. She had a variety of other remedies, some effective like ergot which increases uterine contractions and belladonna which is an antispasmodic, others ineffective. Sneezing powder was often applied as it was believed that sneezing would help dislodge a baby.

The degree of pain a woman suffers in giving birth, and whether it is real or induced by fear, is still a subject of debate today. Yet from the time of Cain, pain has been considered inseparable from childbirth. The Romans called it *poena magna*, the great pain. Although attempts to relieve pain in surgery were made over the centuries using alcohol, opium, Indian hemp or the root of the mandrake, they were not commonly used in childbirth. Christians regarded pain in childbirth as the natural punishment for Eve's sin, and attempts to mitigate it were often condemned. In 1591 Agnes Simpson was burned at the stake for trying to relieve birth pains with opium. However in 1670 in Salem, Massachusetts, Zerobabel Endicott claimed to have found a remedy for 'Sharpe and Difficult Travel in women with child'. His formula was:

> Take a lock of vergins haire on any part of ye head, of half the Age of
> ye woman in travill, cut it very small to fine powder, then take 12
> ant's eggs, dried in an oven after ye bread is drawne, or otherwies
> make them dry and make them to powder with the haire, give this a
> quarter of a pint of red cow's milk or for worst of it give it in strong
> ale wort.[17]

Such dubious remedies apart, in a normal birth the midwife's real value

seems to have been her psychological support, the placebo value of her remedies and her patience and trust in nature.

In addition to the support offered by the attendants there were a wide variety of supernatural aids. Stones in particular have been used as amulets throughout recorded history, and a mediaeval lapidary claimed that the 'jasper helpeth a woman in bering of children and deleverance'.[18] St Hildegard of Bingen, a famous abbess of the eleventh century, recommended a pregnant woman to hold a jasper in her hand for the whole nine months and during the birth because 'the tongue of the ancient serpent extends itself to the sweat of the infant emerging from that mother's womb, and he lies in wait for both mother and infant at the time'.[19]

The eaglestone, apart from preventing abortion and easing delivery, was meant actually to push the unborn child out. It was said to retain this power long after birth, and Nicholas Culpeper, the famous eighteenth-century herbalist, wrote:

> ... the stone aetites held to the priveties is of extraordinary virtues and instantly draws away both child and Afterbirthen, but great care must be taken to remove it presently, or it will draw forth the womb and all.[20]

Manuscripts in roll form, or magic girdles, were attributed with similar powers. Girdles often remained in the same family for generations and were still used in some areas in the nineteenth century. Even the Church, which viewed the reliance on the supernatural in birth with suspicion, sometimes sanctioned its practice. In 1536 the Convent of Bruton was reported to possess 'Our Lady's girdle of Bruton, red silk, which is a solemn relic, sent to women travailing which shall not miscarry in partu'.[21]

The Christian liturgy, too, was used in the birth process, and a pregnant woman might have the Athanasian creed *quicunque vult* said over her three times, or *o infans, siue viuus, siue mortuus, exi foras, quia Christus te uocat ad lucem* (O infant, whether living or dead, come forth because Christ calls you to the light).[22]

During birth women were not restricted to the 'lithotomy' position (lying on the back with the feet up) so favoured by twentieth-century attendants of birth. Indeed, prior to the eighteenth century, women rarely gave birth lying down, and the Hippocratic belief that the baby assisted in its own delivery meant that positions favouring gravity were most popular. Depending on which position she found most comfortable, a woman might squat, kneel, or stand supporting herself with a rope or sheet flung over the rafters, or by leaning against a bench.

The birthing stool, a horseshoe-shaped chair, had been in use since ancient times, and when it was reintroduced from Italy in the fifteenth century it became very popular, particularly in Europe. When a birthing

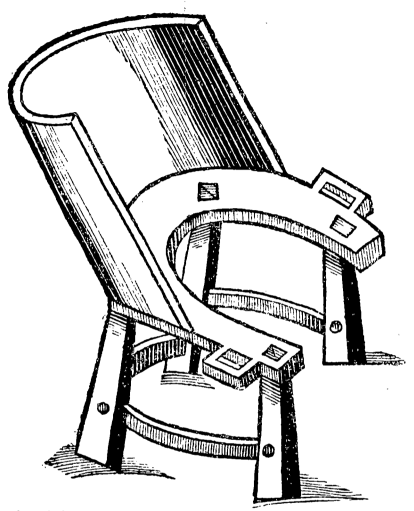

Woodcut of a birthing stool. Such stools have been recorded since the time of the ancient Egyptians, and were popular until the late nineteenth century.

stool was not available, improvisation was often used and either two chairs would be pushed together on which the woman would balance, or the woman might sit on someone's lap.

There were other considerations, too. In Hungary a woman would spend the first part of labour on the bed, but as delivery approached she would leap to the floor or onto a pile of straw because of concern about soiling the sheets. Concern for the bed linen seems to have been quite widespread.

During the late seventeenth century and the eighteenth century it became fashionable to deliver on a bed. It was a move that took hold

25

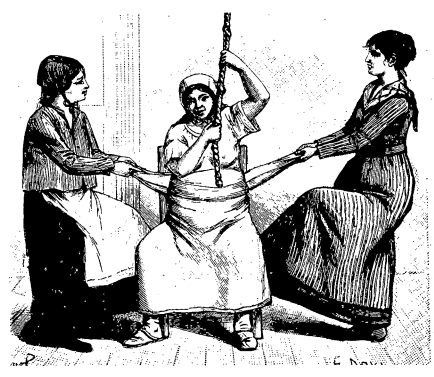

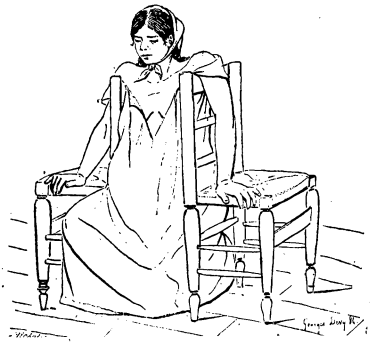

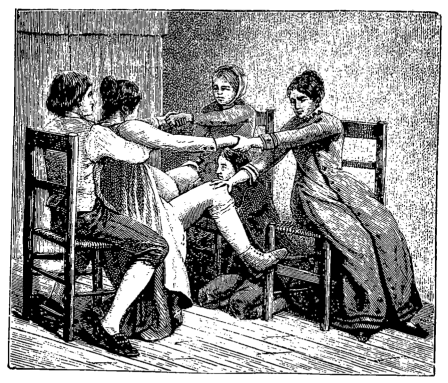

Some of the positions adopted by women for giving birth.

among the British upper classes, and it coincided with the growing importance of the man midwife — indeed is often thought to have been a ploy introduced by men for their own convenience. Percival Willughby, a leading man midwife in the seventeenth century, advocated birth on the bed:

> Let me persuade and intreat the midwife not to torment the poor woman, at the first coming of her pains, by putting her to kneel, or to sit on a woman's lap, or on the midwife's stool, but suffer her to walk gently, or lie down on a truckle bed.[23]

His main concern was the comfort of the woman herself and this was probably the most important factor initially in the move to the bed.

But women who gave birth on a bed were not restricted to it for the whole labour. In the first stage of labour they were allowed to move about, it being accepted that this speeded up delivery; only as the actual delivery approached would the woman lie on the bed. Charles White, a leading man midwife in the eighteenth century, always delivered patients in the horizontal position. He believed that any other position presented the possibility of 'laceration of the perineum and spincter ani, prolapse of

27

the vagina and anus, inversion of the uterus, retention of secundines, flooding, after pains, fainting and even death'.[24]

While most men midwives seem to have concurred that the horizontal position was best, it was women who dictated which position they took on the bed. There were variations from country to country. British and American women favoured lying on the left side near the edge of the bed with the thighs drawn up and the attendant behind. In advanced labour the woman's legs were often separated by a pillow. This became known

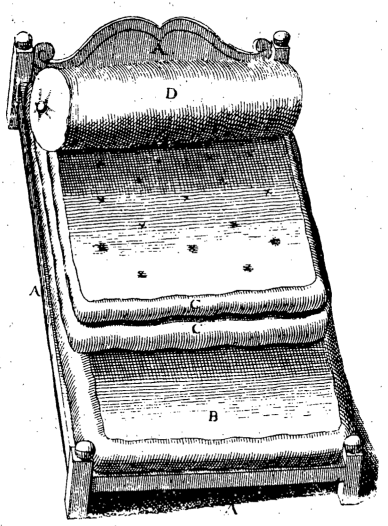

An early delivery bed, showing various positions of the mattress, which could be adjusted for comfort or convenience. (Jacques Mesnard, Le Guide des Accoucheurs, *1743)*

as the 'English position' and was probably adopted for reasons of propriety in that it reduced 'unnecessary exposure'. An American doctor writing in 1867 described this position as 'the almost universal custom' and took the view that it was 'highly inconvenient to the practitioner'.[25] The position had the added advantage, though, of ensuring that a woman could not see what instruments were to be used when intervention was considered necessary.

Interest in the natural position a woman will take in labour is not unique to our times. In his monumental *Histoire des Accouchements*, written in 1891, G J Witkowski devotes a whole section to birthing practices in different races. Although he allows that among primitive people kneeling or squatting seems instinctive, he notes an exception, the woman of the 'Noegele'. When left in a room with a bed, obstetric stool and other articles of furniture, she would succumb, in the final instance to the bed. Like Charles White, Witkowski's conclusion was that the vertical position was best for early labour and the horizontal position for delivery.

Whatever its merits, the British custom of taking to the bed was soon followed by the middle classes in most European countries, although not all women adopted the 'English position'. French women seem to have preferred to lie on their backs, supported by pillows. By the 1840s the pendulum had begun to swing away from the birthing stool. Where once it had been seen as a symbol of progress it was now being discarded because it was 'uncomfortable, looked repellent and put women in a panic. It had become a symbol of pain in childbirth.'[26]

After the birth

After the delivery of the child and placenta there was one immediate concern: baptism. If the baby was very weak and there were fears for its survival, a private baptism was often performed in the home. Indeed, when a delivery showed signs of complications, the baby might be baptised while still inside the uterus. When a foot appeared first, this could immediately be baptised; if a Caesarean was necessary, holy water could be sprinkled on the baby as soon as the uterus had been cut open. Even if all went well baptism usually took place soon after birth, though the mother would not attend as she had not yet been purified.

After the baptism friends and relations would usually gather for a party and, particularly in traditional peasant society, this was often a riotous celebration which could continue for days. This apart the lying-in period was essentially one of quiet and rest. Both midwives and doctors concurred in the belief that bed-rest for nine days — and often considerably longer — was necessary. The mother was made to lie flat on her bed, not moving even when the bed was made. At the end of the

29

nineteenth century, Francis Ramsbotham, a leading obstetrician, recommended that only after two weeks might a woman 'begin to put her feet on the ground'.[27] In fact such inactivity could present a real threat to the mother, allowing blood to coagulate and form clots — an embolism — which could damage her health or kill her.

The length of time women spent resting varied considerably but there are many recorded instances of the belief in the benefit of bed-rest, particularly among the wealthy and aristocracy. In the seventeenth century when Margaret, Duchess of Wemyss, heard from her daughter that she was up and about after fifteen days, she replied in alarm:

> I pray God continue you in health, but it's not the way to be soon very
> well and strong, to try your strength too much. In this cold weather
> your bed had been better for you, I think.[28]

Nearly a century later, in 1792, the physician of Mrs Campbell of Barcaldine imposed a rigid regime. The house was to be kept as quiet as possible for the first week, although Mrs Campbell would be allowed a constant companion to chat to. Each evening she was to be helped into a chair so that her bed could be made. Sheets were to be changed twice a week and night clothes every two days. If she felt like moving she could, so long as there was someone there. Food was to be light but sustaining but, 'she should not by any means venture out of her room before the sixteenth day at soonest'[29] and not outside the house before the twenty-second day. In colonial America, too, the lying-in period was adhered to in order to allow a woman to regain her strength. The female attendants who had gathered for the birth would take charge of onerous household duties and stay for three or four weeks.

Despite the belief in the value of bed-rest such an indulgence was not a possibility for the vast majority of women. A mother might well have to stumble from her bed to prepare the baptismal feast, and almost certainly was up on the second or third day. In 1759 Moritz Thilenius commented:

> . . . you would be astonished to see peasant women going about
> their household tasks that same evening after delivery. I once saw a
> mother, who had delivered the night before, caring for the livestock
> the next day, without paying it any mind.[30]

Ironically, this did at least save such women from the dangers bed-rest could present.

Like the birth itself, the lying-in period was largely a female concern and husbands were little involved. Before a woman had been cleansed by a Ceremony of Purification intercourse was banned. In traditional European society safeguards against contact with the new mother were upheld long after such practices had ceased to be bolstered by religious sanctions. In some areas a woman who had just given birth would be warded off with a broom if she appeared in public and was sometimes forbidden to fetch water from the well because of the fear that she might contaminate it. As long as her husband respected the ban on intercourse this period at least allowed the woman some time to recover physically from the rigours of the birth.

Objections to the 'kirking' or 'churching' ceremony and its association with a woman's loss of grace had been raised by Puritan reformers like John Knox in the sixteenth century. In England in the seventeenth century, when Archbishop Laud attempted to reintroduce the penitential element by insisting on the wearing of a veil or handkerchief for the ceremony, he met with resistance. In 1639, for instance, Dorothy Hazard, wife of a Bristol parson, received women into her house for lying-in so that they could avoid the disagreeable churching ceremonies elsewhere. The ceremony continued to be practised by the Anglican and Catholic churches, however, until the twentieth century, although more as a ceremony of thanksgiving than of marking the removal of a woman's contamination.

HAZARDS OF CHILDBIRTH

> For you ought to know, your death has entered into you and you may
> have conceived that which determines but about nine months at the
> most, for you to live in the world. Preparation for death is that most
> reasonable and most seasonable thing, to which you must now apply
> yourself.[1]

While women accepted the burden of motherhood as their natural lot, they approached birth with trepidation rather than joy. The celebrations that followed a successful birth were a release from the tensions before and during the process. No one doubted that delivery was a painful and dangerous ordeal, and many women would have had relations or friends who had died in childbirth.

There are many records of how the spectre of death haunted pregnant women. In the 1690s, when the Countess of Dalhousie was visiting London and discovered she was pregnant, she wrote home, 'I could wish to be well quit of my big belly in this place, for I am in great fear.'[2] One lady, Elisabeth Josceline, wrote down advice for her children — to obviate the 'loss my little one should have, in wanting me'.[3] Her writing was printed as *The Mother's Legacy to her Unborn Child*, and by 1625 had gone through three editions. It was reprinted unaltered in 1684. Elisabeth dreaded the pain of 'that kind of death', and although she in fact survived the birth she died nine days later and 'was wrapped in that very winding sheet which she had already secretly bought for herself'.[4]

Sarah Stearns, a Massachusetts woman, when about to give birth to her first child, wrote after receiving communion with relatives, 'perhaps this is the last time I shall be permitted to join with my earthly friends'.[5] Such fatalistic attitudes persisted, and as recently as 1914 a working-class woman in England said, 'I always prepared myself to die, and I think this awful depression is common to most at this time.'[6]

Efforts to 'cheat death' through the guidance of omens or the use of amulets were widespread. Even if most births were unhindered by complication, women were acutely aware of the risks involved.

While many might dispute the claim that 95 per cent of births today are without complication,[7] there is plenty of evidence to suggest that this did not hold true in the past. On average complications probably arose in one in ten births,[8] the most common difficulties occurring during delivery. Of course, it is difficult to assess what can be regarded as a 'normal' labour, partly because it is subjective, and partly because attitudes to labour have changed considerably over the centuries.

Today the average length of a first labour is twelve hours. Few labours are allowed to continue for more than twenty hours because of fears for the safety of the child. In the past, the average woman's labour lasted about five hours longer[9] but sometimes considerably more, partly because attendants were less likely to intervene. A protracted labour could last forty-eight hours or more. In most instances the outcome was successful but the longer a woman laboured the more her own health and life were put at risk. As the mother tired she became dehydrated and feverish and the baby began to suffer from lack of oxygen. As a midwife in the American South recounted:

> ... anyone can stand a day of being in labour, it's on the second and third and fourth day when you're 'plum wore out' and 'feel like you can't do nothing else' that you wish you could die and don't see how you can stand it.[10]

Complications

The causes of a long labour are various. It might be that the contractions are weak or the cervix is taking a long time to dilate; the maternal pelvis might be particularly small, or the baby might have a disproportionately large head. The number of children a mother had already had and her age could also influence the length of labour.

The early twenties are usually regarded as the best age for a woman to give birth but this was not always a possibility. The tenuous economics of peasant society meant that there was often not enough property to go round which made it difficult for a young man or woman to set up a separate household and form a family. Many women, particularly in the eighteenth century, did not give birth to their first child until they were in their thirties.[11] As a consequence, labours for such women lasted much longer and instrumental intervention was required much more often.

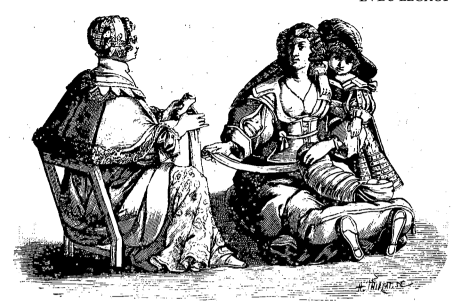

A woman swaddling her baby. (Eighteenth century engraving by Abraham Bosse)

The prevalence of the childhood disease, rickets, was another major cause of complications in delivery.[12] Rickets occur when the bones do not harden properly, and as a result grow crooked, often remaining so for life. The cause is a lack of Vitamin D. Vitamin D allows the absorption of the necessary calcium and phosphorous to make the bones hard. Without it the calcium available in the mother's milk cannot be utilised. It can be supplied by diet, but where this is inadequate, it can be obtained by exposure to sunlight.

This simple remedy, however, was denied many babies, particularly in pre-industrial Europe, partly because of the traditional fear of fresh air and cold, but more importantly because of the custom of swaddling babies for months after birth.

One of the reasons for swaddling which probably began in Roman times was to keep a baby straight and to 'accustom him to keep upon the feet, for else he would go upon all fours as most other animals do'.[13] In fact, the effect was quite the opposite; for swaddling, by excluding sunlight, made rickets the more likely.

When swaddling began to be abandoned during the eighteenth century, rickets continued to be a problem. With industrialisation and the recruitment of children into the labour force, many children spent their lives in factories and seldom saw the light of day. Even when they were not working, the rays of the sun in industrial cities were often obscured by the widespread pollution.

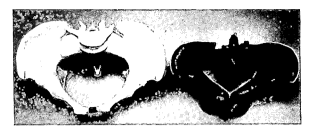

Rickets could have a drastic effect on the pelvis. Left, a normal pelvis. Right, a rachitic pelvis.

Rickets affects both men and women, but it represents a particular danger to women because of the damage it can cause to the construction of the pelvis. A pelvis deformed by rickets might mean that the baby simply cannot pass through unless assisted by instrumental intervention.

Not surprisingly, rickets aroused great fear in women, and in the seventeenth century it was reported that:

> The wild Irish do break the pubic bones of the female infant, so soon as it is born. And I have heard some wandering Irish women affirm the same to be true, and that they have ways of keeping these bones from uniting. It is for certain that they be easily, and soon, delivered. And I have observed that many wanderers of that nation have had a waddling and lamish gesture in their going.[14]

The degree of deformity caused by rickets was very variable but William Smellie, one of the pioneers of midwifery in the eighteenth century who first associated rickets with pelvic anomalies, believed that few women who contracted rickets escaped unaffected:

> Most of those who have been rickety in their infancy, whether they continue little and deformed, or recovering of that disease, grow up to be tall stately women, are commonly narrow and distorted in the pelvis: and consequently subject to tedious and difficult labours.[15]

It has been suggested that up until the 1920s one lower-class, urban woman in four in Europe and America was likely to suffer a delay in labour because of the disease.[16]

Apart from the dangers posed by an overly small pelvis, the greatest fear of a woman in labour was that the baby's head might not descend first. Although such malpresentations affect only a tiny percentage of mothers, they are a very real danger to mother and baby. Breech births, with the feet, knees or buttocks appearing first, can proceed naturally for the mother, although there is an increased risk of injury to the baby because the head is the last part to be born. Far more dangerous for the mother and baby are a face presentation or a transverse lie. In the first case, the baby's face appears first, and because its head is being pushed backward rather than flexed forward it is unable to move. In the second case, because the baby lies across the pelvis, an arm will often appear first, and in such a position the baby cannot be delivered naturally. If the position is not corrected, the mother and baby will die.

Dealing with complications

Although a woman unable to deliver would sometimes be abandoned to her fate, some form of intervention was usually attempted. Much depended, however, on the skill of the attendants. In many areas women depended on untrained midwives or the advice of friends and neighbours. When a complication arose these attendants had little to offer except folkloric remedies or brute force.

Folklore was often based on superstition, and there was considerable regional variety. In Ireland, country people 'loosened every place, person or thing in or about the house, unlocking all the locks ... untying all the knots, even setting free the cows in the byre'[17] if labour was delayed. In parts of Hungary there were more dramatic customs: the husband would step over his wife three times, fumigate her vulvar area by burning the band of his underpants or burning hair from his and his wife's armpit — or, failing this, have intercourse with her.[18] (While this latter would have done nothing to correct a malpresentation, it might have had the effect of speeding up uterine contractions as human semen contains prostaglandin, an oxytocic, or stimulating agent.)

Drugs might also have been administered and some, like ergot — which dramatically increases uterine contractions — and belladonna, could be effective. The difficulty lay in assessing the correct dose; ergot, a powerful agent, might well have caused such an increase in contractions that the uterus ruptured. Other remedies, such as the 'ankle bone of a rabbit which has been shot on one of the first three Fridays in March' or 'a couple of spoonfuls of the water in which two eggs have been cooked'[19] can have done little.

Sometimes the last line of attack would be violent physical action, tossing the woman in a blanket, holding her upside down or shaking her bed. One thing was certain: even if the mother did then deliver, untold harm would almost certainly have been done to her uterus and birth canal.

In certain cases of pelvic contraction or malpresentation, the only means of salvation was manual or instrumental intervention; midwives and relations often preferred to abandon a woman to her fate. Women themselves sometimes elected to die rather than submit to the alternatives. All too frequently manual intervention consisted of pulling on any part of the child and almost always such cases ended in disaster. Neither midwives nor doctors were immune from such practices. One observer of such an instance wrote in 1752: 'If the midwife finds any unusual presentation she becomes confused and ... begins to pull, even if it is a polyp growing to the uterus, whereby often the mother pays with her life.'[20] For attendants who were not trained in anatomy, the temptation to pull was particularly great and had the virtue, from their point of view, of at least demonstrating some form of action to the relations. As a consequence a baby's head or arms could be literally dragged off its body, or even cut off. Percival Willughby records a case in England in 1670. Three midwives having failed to pull out a baby by its arm, cut it off. When Willughby arrived they brought him the baby with the detached arm held to its side by a shirt.

> It was so well done and shrouded that to one who knew nothing and had only looked on the child's body, thus shrouded, this ill work at a distance could not have been perceived that the arm was cut off at the shoulder.[21]

Gruesome as this sounds, the baby would probably have been long since dead, and may have begun to putrefy; it had, in any case, somehow to be removed to save the mother.

Fortunately there was another form of manual intervention that could be of real help to a mother in difficulties — version or turning. This technique was known to the Ancient Greeks and seems to have been used by the more skilled midwives, but it became accepted in medical practice only after the sixteenth century. The main aim of version is to turn the baby from a position where delivery is impossible — a transverse lie — usually to a position where the feet or buttocks present first (podalic version), but sometimes so that the head presents first (cephalic version). The technique sounds very straightforward, but in fact it is not. It involves inserting the hand between contractions, when the cervix is fully dilated and manoeuvring the baby down. It could be extremely dangerous to both mother and child, and it was incredibly painful. Many women had to be tricked into it, preferring to die or risk a Caesarean.

Sometimes version was not possible because the head was wedged so tightly that a hand could not pass it. Then the only recourse was instrumental intervention.

Until the seventeenth century such operations were usually performed by the barber or barber surgeon — only he was supposed to use instruments. The least horrifying of these was the blunt hook which could be used to bring down a baby's thighs in a breech delivery: even this could dislocate or break a baby's thigh. Far more feared were the sharp hooks, crochets, hooked knives and perforators for these were the instruments associated with craniotomy or embryotomy. Although these were probably the most ancient obstetric operations they were regarded with odium because while saving the mother they meant the destruction of the baby.

Embryotomy involved dismembering the baby in order to remove it and craniotomy, piercing the baby's skull and pulling it out with hooks.

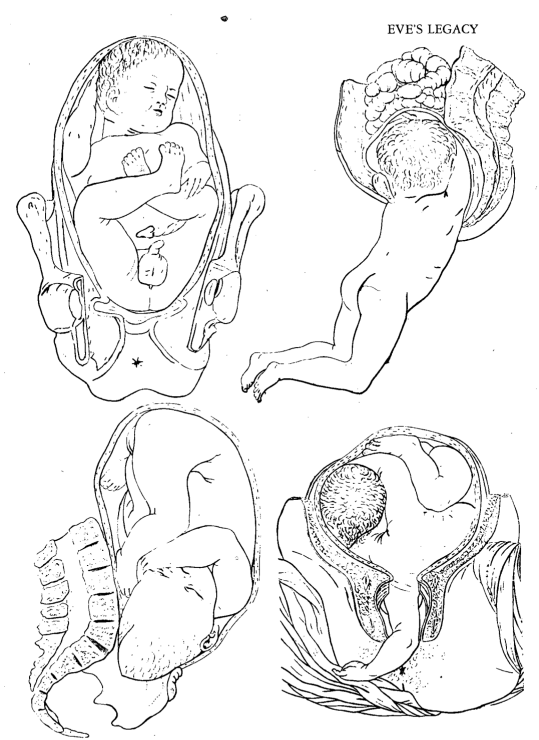

Various forms of malpresentation. Particularly dangerous for the mother and baby was a transverse lie, bottom left.

Although such operations could save the mother, she was often lacerated either by the instruments or by the jagged bits of bone which protruded if the baby's skull had to be crushed.

Despite attempts to restrict the use of instruments to surgeons, midwives too performed these operations. Urban midwives in the Middle Ages always carried an iron hook in case it was necessary to extract a dead baby although they were expected to call in other midwives to ascertain if the baby was dead. In country areas, the operation was sometimes carried out on live babies too, and doctors and untrained midwives might use anything at hand to hook the baby out. Louis Baudeloque, a leading man midwife in France in the eighteenth century claimed 'the midwives and surgeons of the country side, who generally own few instruments, resort for the sake of getting the head out to the iron hooks which the peasants use to suspend their lamps'.[22] Despite their dangers craniotomy and embryotomy were often the only means of dealing with an obstruction and were used in extreme cases until the end of the nineteenth century and beyond.

Although Caesarean section has an equally long history it was fraught with even greater hazards. To reach the baby an incision has to be made in the belly, the connective tissues between the major muscles of the abdomen and the fatty layer beneath cut through and the bladder placed on one side before cutting through the wall of the uterus. Before the days of anaesthesia, the problems of infection in the open abdomen, the shock of pain and the risk of internal bleeding meant that it was usually performed only on mothers who had died. Despite isolated successes, Caesarean section only began to become viable at the end of the nineteenth century.

Before then other techniques to relieve pelvic constriction had been devised — pubiotomy which involved sawing through the pubic bone and symphisiotomy which meant dividing the junction of the two pubic bones. However, to achieve only half an inch of extra space in the diameter of the pelvis the pubic bones needed to be separated by at least two inches. Even when it proved successful in releasing the baby, the mother could be maimed for life, unable to walk or rendered permanently incontinent. Properly performed, symphiosotomy is still used with success today by midwives in remote areas who are unable to call on other surgical aid.

Far more important for mother and surgeon alike was the invention in the seventeenth century of a new tool — the forceps. By the eighteenth century forceps were fast becoming a popular alternative to craniotomy. Forceps are simply a large set of tongs. Each blade can be inserted separately and then locked in place. Variations on the forceps like the filet, a strip of flexible but firm material for hooking round the baby, or the vectis or lever which was like one blade of the forceps, were also used.

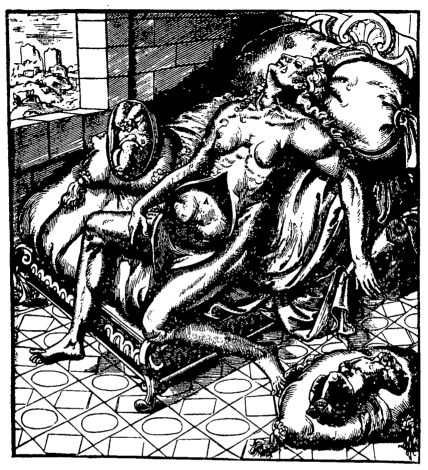

A Caesarean operation showing the baby in utero, *outside the mother's body but still in the membranes, and then after it had been freed from the membranes. (Engraving by Jean Cousin, 1582)*

The great advantage of the forceps was the tremendous leverage it allowed the attendant, with the result that delivery could be effected much more speedily. By the same token terrible damage could be inflicted by the unskilled, particularly if the baby's head had not descended into the pelvis or if the cervix was not dilated. Lisbeth Burger, a midwife, described a birth at which she and the father had to hold down the mother while the doctor performed a forceps delivery:

> The groaning and whimpering of the mother dominated everything in the room, the jerking and shaking of her tortured body ... After all that pulling and levering, holding and bleeding, the child finally emerged from the mother's lap. Torn and haemorrhaging, exhausted to death, the poor mother lay back against the cushions.[23]

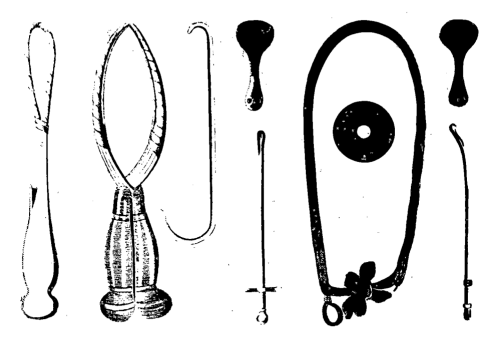

Midwifery instruments such as these were the tools of the man midwife or the barber surgeon.

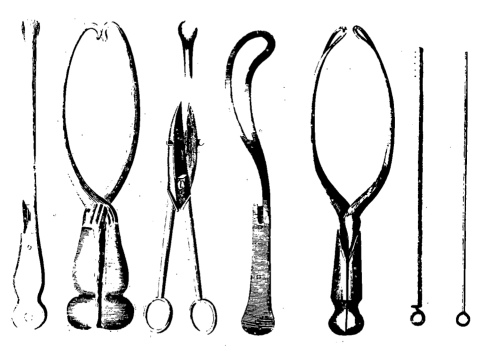

Nor were forceps always successful in delivering the baby, and in such cases the only recourse was usually craniotomy.

Despite the fear of forceps, the ability to terminate long labours was to outweigh the disadvantages of the instrument, and it became one of the most popular tools of birth, normal or abnormal.

Haemorrhage

Even with the safe delivery of her child the dangers to the mother were not over. She could still face danger from haemorrhage or convulsions.

Once the placenta is delivered and following an initial flow of blood, the uterus usually contracts and the blood vessels are closed off. In some instances, however, the uterus does not contract automatically, and then haemorrhage can occur. Haemorrhaging was an ever-present danger. Guillaume De La Motte, a French man midwife, wrote in the early eighteenth century:

> It is only too common to see women perish from blood loss. The number is not small who pay for this accident with their lives after giving birth. During a time when everyone thinks only of rejoicing in the happy delivery of a cherished infant, their strength is running out with their blood, and death arrives gently before one would even have thought it possible.[24]

The causes were many: anaemia, prolonged labour, too many previous deliveries or inept handling of the removal of the placenta. In attempting to remove it, parts of the placenta could remain behind and further efforts to retrieve them could often cause haemorrhage. Sometimes the whole uterus was inverted with the same result.

Until the discovery of ergometrine and the perfection of blood transfusion techniques in the twentieth century, there was little that could be done to stem the flow of blood. There were, however, many folkloric remedies. In Finland a woman's clean shirt was put on a hunting dog which had just returned from the forest. This wet garment would then be drawn over the bleeding woman.[25] Possibly the shock of the cold would have stopped the flow of blood. More realistically, attempts might be made to pad the vagina with warm cloths, or to apply cold or warm douches of water. The greatest successes, prior to transfusions, were achieved with ergot which proved effective in causing the uterus to contract. Ergot was used by some midwives long before it was taken up by the medical profession in the nineteenth century.

In cases of placenta praevia (where the placenta is completely or partly implanted over the cervix so that the baby cannot pass), death from haemorrhage was almost inevitable. In the case of a partially implanted placenta, where there is still room for the cervix to dilate, delivery may be

41

possible. The essential needs are speedy delivery and a particularly skilful attendant, as both mother and child are in real danger. Many urban midwives could and did deal successfully with such cases, but an untrained attendant could rarely cope and the outcome then would be fatal.

Eclampsia

Another ever-present danger was from convulsions or eclampsia, of which Alexander Hamilton, Professor of Midwifery in Edinburgh, wrote in 1781: 'no disease is more dreadful or alarming in appearance.'

The first real symptoms were a swelling of the body tissues, particularly at the wrists and ankles. Then, without warning, a fit would begin from which a woman would often die. In March 1669 Francois Mauriceau, one of the pioneers of midwifery in France, recorded a case.

> I was called in to deliver a woman of twenty-five, in labour with her first child. She had been taken with furious convulsions for a day and a half, losing all consciousness and had almost bitten off her tongue with her teeth.[26]

It has been estimated that these fits occurred perhaps once in every 600 deliveries.[27] In some small communities lifetimes could pass without a case, but midwives certainly knew that they were a possibility.

There was no real remedy for convulsions until the late nineteenth century, when some progress began to be made. Even so, it was only in this century that it became possible properly to control this condition.

Infection

Infection following birth seems to have afflicted women throughout history, and was the final tragedy associated with birth. Although it might begin a few hours after birth, the fever often did not appear until a week later — just when it might have been thought that the dangers were over.

The first signs were usually a high temperature, which might then be followed by a variety of other symptoms.

> ...there is nothing more sudden than the changes in the condition of these women ... In the morning they are cheerful and smiling, and seem to be well, yet they are consumed by fever, pulse rapid, features pale and shrunken, and death is written upon their foreheads. They sink and die without a struggle.[28]

This 'post-delivery sepsis' — or puerperal fever as it was known — was commonly associated with a fever combined with some kind of pain or swelling of the abdomen. Lesser fevers or infections such as 'milk fever' or phlebitis — 'white leg' as it was commonly called — were not regarded as being in any way related. Milk fever, for instance, was thought to be caused by the milk leaving the blood to enter the mother's breasts. In fact, a rise in temperature around the third day would probably be another form of infection, such as endometritis, an infection of the lining of the uterus.

Minor rises in temperature were so common that they were accepted as the norm. It was when infection of the uterus was not localised and spread to the bloodstream and then to the abdominal cavity, the veins of the pelvis or the legs that it became a real threat.

The havoc caused by the spread of infection knows no bounds. When bacteria reached the lining of the abdominal cavity, the peritoneum, peritonitis could occur. When it reached the bloodstream via the infected veins of the uterus, poisonous toxins could be produced, or a blood clot might pass around the body and damage the lungs. When the connective tissue of the pelvis was infected, cellulitis could occur and large pockets of pus or abscesses form.

Often more than one of these infections overlapped with another, but because one would appear in a more marked way, that infection would be diagnosed. It has been suggested that virtually all infections recorded in the month after birth may have related to post-delivery sepsis. So in addition to the records of puerperal fever one should add cases recorded as pneumonia, gastric fever, pleuritis, erysipelas and scarlet fever.[29]

The pain and misery involved in most of these infections was terrible. The pain produced by peritonitis, for example, was so severe that one French doctor in the Hotel Dieu in eighteenth-century Paris could diagnose cases by the sharp cry of the woman alone.[30] Often the abdomen was so tender that sufferers could not even stand the pressure of a sheet. Moreover, when women did recover, such infections seriously undermined their subsequent health. A gynaecology textbook of the 1880s asserted: 'It is the rare exception to examine a multiparous female pelvis without finding some traces of a previous cellulitis or peritonitis.'[31] These traces, either abscesses, adhesions or chronic tubal infections, were 'an enduring painful souvenir of her infection. A bloodstream infection that does not produce great buckets of pus may, on the other hand, leave a different souvenir: a permanently damaged heart or kidney disease.'[32]

The lying-in hospitals founded in the seventeenth and eighteenth centuries — supposedly for the relief of women in childbirth — were, in fact, to prove breeding grounds for the fever. Some of these hospitals subjected women to probably the most septic environments anywhere. One description of the Hotel Dieu in Paris in 1788 conjures up a grim picture. Huge beds were crammed into the wards which had

> . . . little alleys and dim passageways among them, where the walls

> are covered with spittle, the floor covered by the filth that drains
> from the mattresses and from the commodes when they're emptied,
> as well as with the pus and blood that pour down from wounds or
> bloodlettings.[33]

Infected and healthy mothers shared the same bed, often in the same room as terminal venereal disease cases, in wards right on top of the morgue and with the hospital's dirty laundry in a chest at the end of the delivery. Following such a description, it is little wonder that the conclusion was that 'in no place in Europe, in no city, in no village, in no hospital, nowhere is the loss of new mothers comparable to that of the Hotel Dieu of Paris'.[34]

It was only at the end of the eighteenth century that the fever began to be understood. Even then, it was not until the mid-nineteenth century that preventive measures began to be taken, and not until the discovery of bacteria and the introduction of antiseptics at the end of the century that mortality began to fall. In the meantime, puerperal fever continued to haunt women in all walks of life.

RISING EXPECTATIONS

> It is no exaggeration to say that for centuries women's lives had been
> overshadowed by the burden of childbearing, their whole attitude to
> life affected by the knowledge that they would probably spend their
> fertile years in a succession of pregnancies culminating each time in
> a painful and life-threatening labour. At long last, however, this
> suffering was to be alleviated.[1]

At last during the nineteenth century the rapid growth of the sciences made medicine really effective for the first time. In particular a number of breakthroughs had a direct bearing on women in childbirth and were to eliminate many of the hazards they had faced before.

It has been suggested that these developments were accompanied by a declining sense of fatalism on the part of middle-class Victorian women, that they no longer regarded pain and death as uncontrollable aspects of existence and felt that they should and could be conquered.[2] Yet medical advance and women's aspirations did not develop in tandem — in part because of the time lag between medical invention and its application, but also because new notions of modesty and morality engulfed the Victorian middle class as never before and prevented women from taking full advantage of what was available.

The constraints imposed on middle-class women were reinforced by a general decline in their health. When in 1855 Catherine Beecher, an American hygienist, conducted a survey of women's health, she concluded that good health was so rare that many women did not know what it was like. Middle-class women seemed to suffer greater pain, to be more nervous and generally less healthy than their mothers or grandmothers.

The new standards of the middle-class lifestyle imposed strains on women. They were anxious to maintain zealously the cleanliness of the home, but for lower middle-class women who had little help in the home their work was very taxing.

Even when they had plenty of servants, women spent most of their lives in unaired and dark houses where any vents were blocked to conserve heat, and curtains were usually drawn to avoid damage to the furniture. Cocooned in their homes they were exposed to noxious fumes from coal that had no means of escape. It was only towards the end of the century that the health of these women began to show any real improvement, probably because of higher living standards and warmer, cleaner and less crowded homes.

The frailty of women's health lent credence to the notion that women, unlike men, were ruled by their emotions, and that this affected their health:

> . . . there is another aspect of most material consequence to the health of the female . . . I mean the due regulation of her mental constitution, and her moral feelings and affections . . . To what use is it carefully to observe the external and physical laws of health, if in herself she raises an agent more powerful to subvert her health than they are to preserve it? The influence of strong or violent mental emotion, whether exciting — as of joy, hope, anger, or rage; or depressing as of fear and despair we well know to suppress a powerful and immediate influence over the vital functions. Death has often followed instantaneously.[3]

Not everyone subscribed to such extreme views, of course, but women were increasingly considered unfit for life in the outside world. Any venture into it was likely to 'unsex' them and render them incapable of fulfilling their roles as wives and mothers. Romantic novels, cards and late nights were discouraged.

The dictates of women's fashion, and the corset in particular, were also blamed for causing women real physical damage. 'Lacing in' of garments began among the aristocracy about the eleventh or twelfth centuries. Gradually the practice filtered down to middle-class women. By the mid-nineteenth century, when the fifteen or eighteen inch waist was the ideal, physicians were attributing to the constrictions of the corset a litany of devastating consequences. In addition to making birth more difficult it was believed to cause spinal deformities, tuberculosis, all kinds of internal bleeding, fainting, diarrhoea and anal prolapse.

Recently it has been argued that many of the ills were credited to the corset because doctors' knowledge of how the body works was deficient:

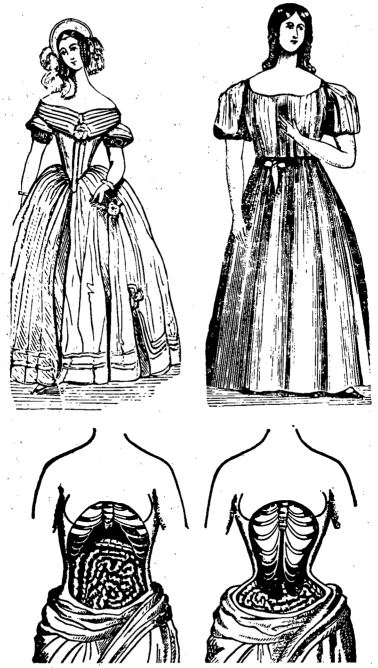

The natural position of a woman's organs, and how they were believed to be distorted by the wearing of corsets. (B Grant Jefferies and J L Nichols, Searchlight on Health: Light on Dark Corners 1904)

... the only injury that can reliably be attributed to tight lacing is
'hiatus hernia' in which a portion of the stomach slides into the
lower abdomen. The other symptoms were probably all either
coincidence or the work of overactive medical imaginations.[4]

Whatever the truth it contributed to the widespread concern for women's
health. The nineteenth century saw a spate of books on the subject and a
plethora of non-surgical crazes. Everything from electricity and massage
to medicated tampons, paste and medicines was advocated. In 1867, a
Doctor W H Buck declared it 'outrageous' that some doctors were making
the vagina a 'Chinese toy shop' filled with mechanisms. Whereas 'our
grandmothers never knew they had a uterus until it was filled with a
healthy fetus', even young women had to have their 'wombs shored up
with a pessary'. He claimed there were 123 kinds of mechanism available,
'from a simple plug to a patent threshing machine, which can only be
worn with the largest hoop'.[5]

The popular health movement, which was particularly widespread in
America, fostered the new concern for health. As the century progressed
lay people became increasingly interested in the workings of their own
bodies and were encouraged to develop healthy habits — excercise,
moderate diet, plenty of fresh air, unrestricted clothing and regular baths.
Men and women attended public lectures on physiology, and the 'Ladies
Physiological Societies' were the backbone of the movement. Women
were admonished to know and to be able to control their own bodies; this
led many women to demand less painful birth, and encouraged the
limitation of families.

Particular concern was shown in respect of childbirth; the ideal of
motherhood was given a greater prominence and almost all married
women experienced pregnancy once and often four or five times. Most
middle-class women married between twenty and twenty-six so, at least
in the first half of the century, more than a quarter of their lives were
spent in pregnancy or in nursing and recovery from birth. A huge market
in women's magazines developed and some of the articles in these reveal
their anxieties:

> No-one who has reflected upon the subject, and certainly no-one
> who has a practical acquaintance with it, will contend that the annual
> deaths of 3,000 women in childbirth, and of 13,350 boys and 9,740
> girls in the first month after delivery, or the suffering and deformity
> of those who escape with life, are natural and inevitable. Admit that
> the lives of a thousand, or even a hundred — or of one hundred of
> those mothers could be saved — and that many more might be
> rescued from injuries and pains which disable, or never leave them;
> and assuredly, no apathy, no false sentiment of delicacy, will prevent
> those who have the public health at heart from giving the subject the
> most attentive consideration.[6]

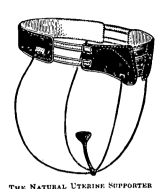

THE NATURAL UTERINE SUPPORTER

THE NATURAL UTERINE SUPPORTER APPLIED.

DR. McINTOSH'S Natural Uterine Supporter.

An advertising circular from Chigaco, c. 1881.

There was a flood of advice to deal with these anxieties. In 1837 Thomas Bull published the first book devoted to antenatal care, *Hints to Mothers for the Management of Health during the Period of Pregnancy and in the lying-in room with an exposure of Common Errors in connection with these subjects.* The chapters covered diet, longings, regulation of the bowels, exercise, dress, care of the breasts and 'The supposed influence of the imagination of the mother upon the child in the womb':

> Why should we be surprised at some irregularities on the skin and other parts of the human body since we see the same thing occurring daily throughout the animal and vegetable world? They have their moles, their discolourations, their excrescenses, their unnatural shapes which it would be very philosophical to ascribe to any effort of the imagination.[7]

The book went to twenty-five editions, indication enough of its popularity. Advice in the birth manuals emphasised the responsibility of the mother for her own health and that of her baby. The importance of early diagnosis was stressed but often the means of ascertaining pregnancy were shunned because of the constraints of modesty.

By the mid-century most middle-class women were using doctors during childbirth in preference to midwives. Doctors had at least some training, they could use obstetrical instruments and seem to have given women a greater sense of security. One report, admittedly by a male doctor, claimed

> I never knew a woman who attended by a medical practitioner who on any future parturition would admit a midwife. I have often heard

women remark how very differently they were treated by their female and their medical attendants; and that females are much more unfeeling than those of the other sex.[8]

Yet doctors were severely curtailed in their behaviour and had built up rituals of examination which allowed them only limited activity. The woman remained fully clothed throughout examination and the doctor would gaze directly into her eyes as an assurance that her private parts were free from his gaze. In Britain and America, even this limited form of investigation — known as 'the touch' — often only took place once labour had begun. The birth was frequently conducted under a sheet to shield the genitalia from view, and it was felt that doctors who could not operate within these restrictions were incompetent.

One of the arch proponents of conservatism in the mid-nineteenth century was Charles Meigs of the Jefferson Medical School in Philadelphia. He was happy to embrace the strictures placed on medicine generally by modesty.

It is, perhaps, best upon the whole, that this great degree of modesty should exist even to the extent of putting a bar to researches, without which no very clear and understandable notions can be obtained of the sexual disorders. I confess I am proud to say that, in this country generally, certainly in my part of it, there are women who suffer the extremity of danger and pain rather than waive those scruples of delicacy which prevent their maladies from being fully exposed . . .[9]

As a result many medical advances that could have been of benefit to women were not implemented. In 1836 J M Jacquemier discovered that a change in the colour of the vagina was a useful symptom of early pregnancy. Ascertaining this colour change involved only a simple examination but it was not mentioned in health care manuals until the 1880s. The vaginal speculum, a useful tool in determining the precise condition of pregnancy, was reintroduced during the nineteenth century. It was widely used in France but in Britain it was shunned because of the degree of exposure involved. Some of the loudest and certainly most extreme objections came from doctors:

. . . no one who has realised the amount of moral evil wrought in girls . . . whose prurient desires have been increased by Indian hemp and partially gratified by medical manipulation, can deny that the remedy is worse than the disease. I have . . . seen young unmarried women, of the middle class of society, reduced by the constant use of the speculum, to the mental and moral condition of prostitutes, seeking to give themselves the same indulgence by the practice of solitary vice, and asking every medical practitioner . . . to institute an examination of the sexual organs.[10]

Similarly the stethoscope, which when applied to the woman's stomach

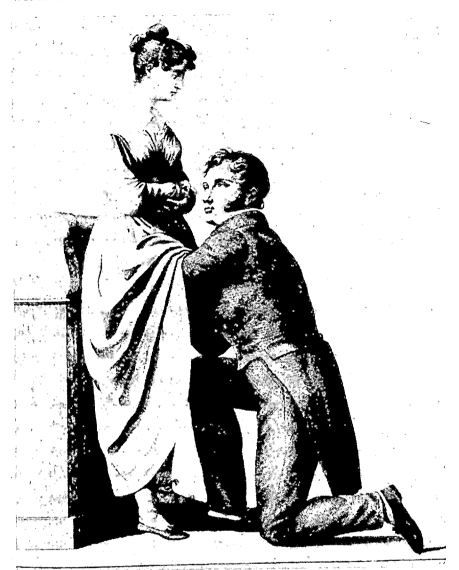

'The Touch', from a popular nineteenth century gynaecological textbook. The
doctor averts his eyes and the woman remains fully clothed. (Jacques-Pierre
Maygriere, Nouvelle Démonstrations d'Accouchemens, 1822.)

could reveal the pattern of the fetal heartbeat and indicate its well-being,
was regarded as indecent. Professor James Hamilton, Professor of
Midwifery in Edinburgh in the first half of the nineteenth century,
questioned Robert Collins, Master of the Rotunda in Dublin, if he
proposed 'to apply the stethoscope to the naked belly of a woman for, if

so, he may be assured that in this part of the world at least, such a proposal would be indignantly rejected by every young or old practitioner of reputed respectability'.[11] Even as late as the 1860s Francis Ramsbotham dismissed the stethoscope on the somewhat flimsy excuse that 'he had no personal experience of using the stethoscope for this purpose'.[12]

The whole question of pain in childbirth was one that exercised the Victorians too. Arguments about it in physiology manuals and women's handbooks demonstrate the same ambivalence as about women's sexuality. To suffer pain was to be feminine, because weakness and sickness were inherent to the female of the species. But not all women suffered. Popular stereotypes were presented to show that childbirth need not be painful — in particular there was the example of the Indian Squaw, the unspoiled child of nature. Her pregnancy, it was asserted, required no special attention or worry and she performed her daily tasks up to the point of labour. She would then give birth on her own and resumed her everyday life almost immediately.

Civilisation was blamed for causing women to feel pain, and many men argued that women suffered because they were no longer truly feminine. They were 'sexually aggressive, intellectually ambitious, and defective in proper womanly submission and selflessness'. The palliative was the return of woman to her properly subordinate, non-aggressive role in the home.[13]

However, moral and medical expectations of women may themselves have given rise to much of the anxiety and fear about birth felt by women and increased the likelihood of pain — a pain which many American doctors described as one of the worst agonies known to them, greater than the terrible suffering experienced by soldiers during the Civil War.

One thing is certain, however, unlike their reactions to other medical innovations, women showed no reluctance to use chloroform. James Young Simpson, Professor of Midwifery in Edinburgh, who first used the drug for childbirth, stated: 'Obstetricians may oppose it, but I believe our own patients themselves will force the use of it upon the profession.'[14] Women could not have had a more stalwart champion than Simpson. He fundamentally believed that:

> If the object of the medical practitioner is really twofold as it has always, until of late been declared to be, *viz*: 'the alleviation of human suffering and the preservation of human life' then it is our duty, as well as our privilege to use all legitimate means to mitigate and remove the physical sufferings of the mother during parturition.[15]

Simpson would use about an ounce of the drug an hour, beginning when the pains became bad towards the end of the first stage, withdrawing it in the intervals when there was no pain. As the baby's head began to pass over the mother's perineum he would increase the dose.

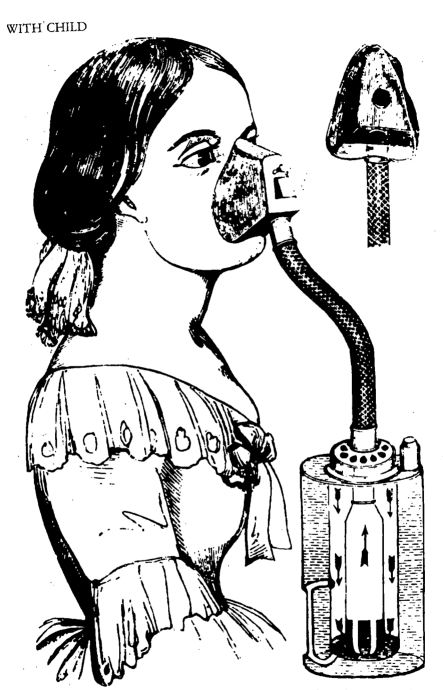

Chloroform masks such as these helped to ensure that the correct dose of chloroform was given, but even when expertly administered chloroform presented dangers because of its toxic effects. (Robert Margota, Illustrated History of Medicine, 1968.)

In America, Simpson's counterpart was Walter Channing, Professor of Midwifery at Harvard. He first used ether to alleviate pains in difficult births but then began to use it for normal labours too, and in 1848 he described the technique he used in his *A Treatise of Etherization in Childbirth*. He challenged doubters to witness the serenity, pleasure and joy produced by ether and compare it with the agony, wretchedness and fear otherwise involved. Yet, particularly in America, many doctors did not use it:

> One great reason for the aversion to child-bearing is the thousand disagreeable and painful experiences which attend the long months of patient waiting, and the certain agony at the end — agony which the tenderest susceptibilities and sympathies of the noblest physician can but faintly imagine — agony which, in not one case in a hundred is mitigated by anaesthesia. If the blessed, benevolent suggestion of the use of the chloroform could be adopted, the world would hear less of abortions.[16]

When it was used it was often only for first births and then only intermittently until just before the child was born. Most doctors regarded this as the time when the most pain was incurred — while, in fact, the most painful time is usually when the cervix is dilating during the first stage of labour.

The objections to pain relief in childbirth were largely based on moral or religious grounds. The religious regarded anaesthesia as a 'decoy of Satan' which 'robbed God of the earnest cries which arise in time of trouble for help'. Simpson, however, was quick to point out that when God removed Adam's rib he caused a deep sleep to fall on Adam which was proof of the Lord's approval. When a Dr Samuel Ashwell took up this point in the *Lancet* and argued that this deep sleep took place before the fall of man and the introduction of pain, Simpson riposted:

> If you refuse to interfere with a natural function because it is natural, why do you ride my dear doctor? You ought to walk, in order to be consistent. Chloroform does nothing but save pain, you allege. A carriage does nothing but save fatigue. Which is more important to be done away with? Your fatigue or your patient's screams and tortures?[17]

Simpson also inquired if the doctor wore clothes — a most unnatural habit!

Religious argument apart, some doctors still regarded anaesthesia as unnatural and even as a breach of medical ethics. Dr Petrie, a Liverpool doctor, felt it was the act of a coward to avoid pain, and if a woman insisted on having chloroform she should be told that she was not fit to make such a decision. 'Are we going to allow the patient to tell us what to do?'[18]

In America, the Philadelphian Dr Meigs opposed the use of anaesthesia on the grounds that 'the very suffering which a woman undergoes in labour is one of the strongest elements in the love she bears for her offspring'. He regarded pain as 'a desirable, salutory and conservative manifestation of the life force',[19] and particularly necessary in an instrumental delivery. If there was no pain how could the doctor be guided in his use of instruments?

Simpson's fighting defence . systematically knocked down his opponents' objections. He advocated that chloroform be made available to every woman in childbirth and waged war by endless letters, papers, pamphlets and lectures. He went on using chloroform, encouraged others to do likewise and instructed his students to use it. His campaign was greatly helped when Queen Victoria used chloroform for the birth of Prince Leopold in 1853. Many doctors were nevertheless genuinely concerned about the growing number of deaths that occurred in surgery where anaesthetics were used. Although many of these deaths were probably caused by the introduction of experimental procedures, chloroform was certainly not an ideal drug. Still, Simpson's fight was a milestone in the development of childbirth: it established a woman's right to pain relief, and was widely accepted by the beginning of the twentieth century.

The greatest obstacle to women's hopes of improved childbirth was the continuing toll of death taken by puerperal fever. It was the single, most common cause of death in childbirth. Ironically, a disproportionate number of casualties was from the middle class. Middle-class women had increasingly turned to doctors to provide better measures for their own health and that of their children but because doctors were more inclined to intervene instrumentally in birth and because a doctor came into contact with a wider variety of infectious diseases in his practice, there was a higher risk of his passing on infection.

Preventive measures to control the spread of infection were known by the 1860s, but many doctors did not implement them. There was considerable resistance to the notion that doctors, 'the healers', were the means of contagion. Although the fever was often difficult to recognise and could be extraordinarily persistent, preventive measures where these were adopted had a dramatic effect on the incidence of the fever. But it was only after the identification of the bacteria that caused the infection in 1879 and after the widespread adoption of antiseptic measures in the late nineteenth century that the fever began to be controlled.

In Britain no significant improvements in maternal mortality can be detected between the beginning of the century and the end. In 1838 the rate was five to every 1,000 births: in 1892 the rate was 4.9 to every 1,000 births.[20] It was only in the last two decades of the century that the number of deaths owing to accidents of birth began to fall. By then medical invention had begun to catch up with medical practice. The introduction of antiseptics and discoveries in bacteriology made puerperal fever less of a danger, and Caesarean section at last became a viable operation.

Taking the century as a whole, however, it can hardly be said that the middle-class woman's hopes had been realised. Pain and possible death did not decrease until the end of the century. Ignorance on the part of some doctors encouraged the tendency to downgrade physical changes and stressed instead the emotional aspects of womankind. The new responsibilities society placed on motherhood seem only to have increased the anxieties of women who, because of their weak physical constitution, were considered particularly unfit to be mothers. Women turned to doctors for improvements; but many could offer only an ambivalent response.

WHO HELPED DELIVER?

It is hardly too much to say that midwives must have begun nine
months after there were two women and one man on earth.
   Sir Francis Champneys, Presidential Address to the Obstetrical
Society, 1895.

See the whole pack open in full cry: to arms! to arms! is the word; and
what are those arms by which they maintain themselves, but those
instruments, those weapons of death!
   Elizabeth Nihell, quoted in Harvey Graham, *Eternal Eve* p159.

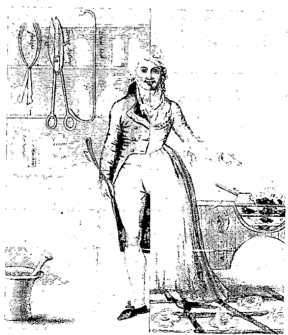

*Cartoon of a man midwife – possibly William Smellie, who was forced on
occasion to don women's clothes to conceal his instruments from his patient.
The shelf with bottles held the potions the man midwife supposedly used to
stimulate desire in his patients. (John Blunt, Man Midwifery Dissected, 1793)*

THE TRADITIONAL MIDWIFE

To aid the labouring woman and to offer her comfort and support, the midwife (literally 'with-wife') has been an established figure throughout recorded history. Until the end of the nineteenth century the majority of babies in Europe and North America were still delivered by women; but with the rise of the medical man during the nineteenth century the position of the midwife was so severely eroded that she ceased to be considered a competent attendant.

Male domination in the birth process is an issue of concern for many women today, so it is important to understand why the competence of the midwife began to be questioned and why, rightly or wrongly, women began to turn to men midwives and doctors for a better quality of care.

As early as 800 BC an Athenian law laid down certain ground rules for midwives, and divided them into two groups — the ordinary midwives who could conduct a normal birth, and the senior or 'doctor' midwives who were called in if there was a complication. These midwives could prescribe drugs, induce abortion or speed up labour. Their knowledge was based on experience rather than any special training; and the techniques they used were age-old too — for example, binding the woman's abdomen with a cloth which was tightened with each pain to help ease out the baby.

A number of Greek and Roman physicians wrote on the subject of childbirth — one of the most important treatises on obstetrics was produced by a physician, Soranus of Ephesus — but it was accepted that the actual birth would be conducted by women. Midwifery was considered to be beneath the dignity of the physician, and certainly the midwife knew far more than he did about the female reproductive organs. As in other ancient societies, though, the physician might be called in for an emergency or if any destructive surgery was needed.

During the Middle Ages, the misogyny of the Church and the taboos surrounding the actual birth meant that the position of the midwife was secure. Because the dissection of corpses was forbidden, surgery was performed only by sow gelders or barbers. So for several centuries the knowledge of the birth process, female anatomy and methods of facilitating labour were accumulated entirely by women. Around the thirteenth century, there is evidence from Germany of the ancient two-tier system of midwifery emerging again in the form of trained urban midwives and their usually untrained and often totally illiterate rural counterparts.

The urban midwife corps was usually headed by a mother superior who had under her control female midwife inspectors who were used to help the salaried town midwife if she ran into trouble. The chief midwife's role was an honorary one, but other midwives were paid fully or partially by the city. Numbers were firmly controlled and regular midwives often had a trainee who served an apprenticeship of a number of years before becoming a midwife herself.[1] These midwives were certainly more knowledgeable and competent than doctors, not only because men were excluded from the birthing chamber, but also because medicine was still limited to the scientific knowledge of Greece and Rome. While for most doctors in the mediaeval period 'obstetrics was a defiling activity, and textbook knowledge was still contaminated with useless mumbo jumbo,'[2] the urban midwife had the benefit of experience. She could cope with an umbilical cord that appeared before the baby, was aware of the effect of ergot in speeding up a slow labour, and probably knew how to perform version when there was a malpresentation.[3] Such midwives were able and willing to hand on their knowledge to other midwives, but they kept it a closely guarded secret from doctors. They felt their knowledge was special and to be used for the greater good of their patients.

The lowly position accorded to midwifery by the Church ensured female domination of the birth chamber but did not exempt it from interference by the Church. The midwife's religious beliefs were a matter of real concern. Because it was part of Christian doctrine that a baby who died unbaptised would not achieve salvation, the Synod of Triers in 1277 ordered priests to instruct lay women in the words of an emergency baptism so that they could carry it out if the priest was not available.[4] Nor was baptism the only reason for the Church's scrutiny of midwives. Childbirth was regarded as a fertile ground for the workings of supernatural forces and the umbilical cord, a caul, the placenta and a stillborn child were believed to play an important part in the rites of witchcraft. Two members of the German Inquisition, for example, claimed that no one did more harm to Catholicism than midwives, 'who surpass all other witches in their crimes'. There are records of cases where midwives were executed for supposedly killing babies and dedicating their souls to the devil.[5]

In some places midwives were required to take a formal oath not to shield the mother who fell short of the Church's standards of chastity, and not to conceal a birth or destroy a child. The first known oath dates from Regensburg in 1452. Midwives were also urged to report the birth of unnatural children, which were considered an indication of liaison with the devil.[6]

As the power of the Church began to wane, supervision of midwives began to pass more and more to municipal authorities. Under this system character references were still important, but much more attention was paid to technical competence. Midwives starting to practice were formally examined by physicians or experienced midwives. This ensured a greater degree of ability, but it also imposed limits on the midwife's scope. Most regulations required the attendance of a doctor or a surgeon in difficult cases.

During the Middle Ages obstetrical literature was virtually non-existent, except for translations into Latin of the work of Greek physicians such as Hippocrates. In the twelfth century a text, *De Passionibus Mulierum Curandarum*, devoted to gynaecology and the affairs of women and attributed to Trotula, was produced in Salerno in Italy. It had little new to add and its advice was limited mainly to the relative efficacy of rival charms and incantations and other dubious recommendations.

In the late fourteenth and fifteenth century, a spate of medical treatises appeared which were written in the vernacular for the first time. A number of these were devoted to childbirth and women's diseases. One of the earliest, a manuscript now known as Sloane 2463, strongly reaffirmed the right of women to be cared for by women:

> And although women have various maladies and more terrible
> sicknesses than any man knows, as I said, they are ashamed for fear
> of reproof in times to come and of exposure by discourteous men
> who love women only for physical pleasure and for evil gratification.
> And if women are sick such men despise them and fail to realise how
> much sickness women have before they bring them into the world.
> And so, to assist women, I intend to write of how to help their secret
> maladies so that one woman may aid another in her illness and not
> divulge her secrets to such discourteous men.[7]

Most of the remedies in Sloane are recipes handed down from classical times, but the manuscript does contain the first account of an operation to repair a ruptured perineum to appear in any treatise on midwifery: after replacing the uterus, and washing the wound with wine and butter, the midwife is instructed to

> sew up the breach . . . in three or four places with a double silken
> thread. Then put a linen cloth into the part, that is to say the vulva,
> according to its size. And afterward cover it with hot tar, and that
> will make the womb withdraw and thus remain firm because of the
> evil smell of the tar, and then the breach will be healed and closed
> with powder of comfrey, little daisy, and cinammon.[8]

Afterwards the woman was to be kept in bed for between seven and nine days, to eat and drink little, and to avoid cold and coughing. The advice was perfectly sound and was probably added at a later stage, but it was many years before it was heeded.

The other points of interest in Sloane and many other such manuscripts were the illustrations of unnatural presentations. Sloane contains sixteen, in which the neck of the womb is shown as little more than a flask shape with a wide neck and with no sign of the placenta or umbilical cord. The child, looking oddly adult, stands inside. These illustrations can have been of little practical help but the instructions on how to cope with such presentations are remarkable for their detail.

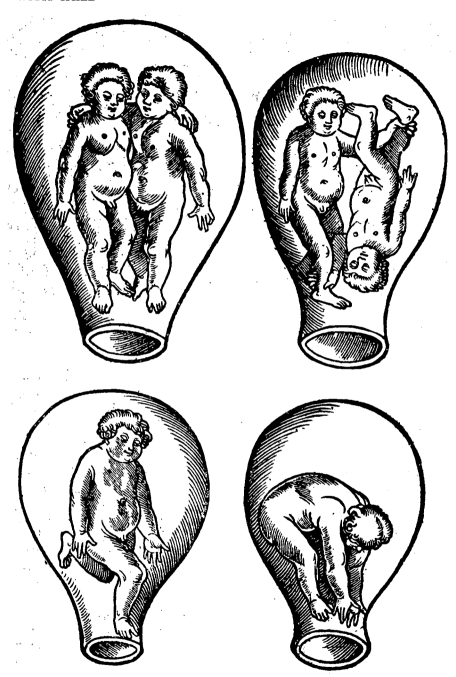

Simplified diagrams of a child in utero *such as these accompanied many of the early midwifery texts, including Sloane 2463.*

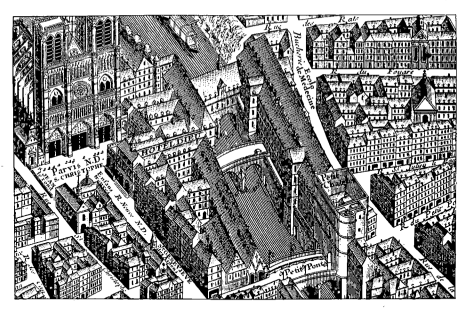

The Hotel Dieu, the famous French hospital which became one of the most important training centres for midwifery. (Plan by Turgot from H Carrier, Origins of the Maternité)

The development of printing in the mid-fifteenth century facilitated publication of a number of books on midwifery. In fact, they offered little more than a perpetuation of ancient traditions, but they formed the basis of most textbooks for midwives until the seventeenth century. By far the most popular was Rosslin's *A Rosegarden for Pregnant Women and Midwives*,[9] published in 1513 in Germany. By 1568 it had been reprinted ten times and translated into Dutch, Czech, French, Danish, Latin and English. The first English edition was translated by Richard Jonas and dedicated to Catherine Howard, wife of Henry VIII. Henry's previous wife, Jane Seymour, had died of puerperal fever. In 1545 the book was enlarged by Thomas Raynalde and renamed *The Birth of Mankynde*. It strongly advocated the use of the birthing stool which was widely used by midwives in Europe and, less frequently, in Britain and America, for the next two centuries. Based mainly on Rosslin's book, it is a mixture of truths and absurdities, and has little scientific merit — though it was regarded as an authoritative treatise on obstetrics for many years.

There were many imitators of Rosslin's book, and although their aim was to benefit the midwife — Thomas Raynalde believed his book would be available to 'the simplest mydwyfe . . . for her better instruction and also other women that have needed for her helpe'[10] — they can in fact have been of little value to the majority of midwives, who would have been illiterate. Far more effective than books for the training of midwives were the schools. One of the first was the Hotel Dieu in Paris, an ancient monastic foundation which began in the sixteenth century to instruct midwives. In the tradition of religious foundations it was a charity, and anyone was accepted for delivery. The names of patients were recorded but never divulged, and many of the children born there were illegitimate. By the second half of the seventeenth century the school was renowned throughout Europe.

One of the earliest pupils at the Hotel Dieu was Louise Bourgeois, who was to become the first great woman practitioner of obstetrics. She practised, trained other women and wrote three books. Louise was married to a barber-surgeon who had been trained by one of the outstanding surgeons of the period, Ambroise Paré. Initially she was instructed by both her husband and Paré then, after attending the Hotel Dieu, she went on to become the sworn midwife of the city of Paris and replaced the official royal midwife, Madame Dupuis. Her first attendance on the queen, Marie de Medici, was in 1601 at Fontainebleau for the queen's first child. The birth was attended by 200 people. Labour was slow, and when the baby was born late in the evening it was distressed. Louise gave the baby wine, which she took in her own mouth and then blew into his throat.

The queen's fourth birth was a breech presentation. The king, Henri IV, said to Louise:

> Sage femme, I know that you hold the life of my wife and of her child
> more dear than your own; do as you would to your own. If you see
> that there is any danger, you know that this man of Paris, who
> delivers women, is here, and he will wait in the grand cabinet.[11]

The man referred to was Honoré, who is said to have been the first man midwife to assist at confinements other than emergencies. Louise did not need to summon him.

Apart from her practice, Louise achieved fame through her midwifery texts. *Observations Diverses* was widely translated, and her published account of Marie de Medici's lyings-in reveal her sense of ethics and the dignity of her profession:

> Undertake, till the last day of your life, to learn; which to do requires
> a great humbleness, for the proud do not win the hearts of those who
> know secrets. Never in your life venture to employ any medicine in
> which you have been instructed, neither on the poor nor on the rich,
> unless you are certain of its virtue and that it can do no harm,
> whether taken within the body or applied upon it. Nor hide the
> medicines you know of from physicians or midwives, lest these be as
> little regarded as the charlatans who employ their medicines alike on
> every occasion, and yet claim to know wonders, and in all they do,
> hide their practise.[12]

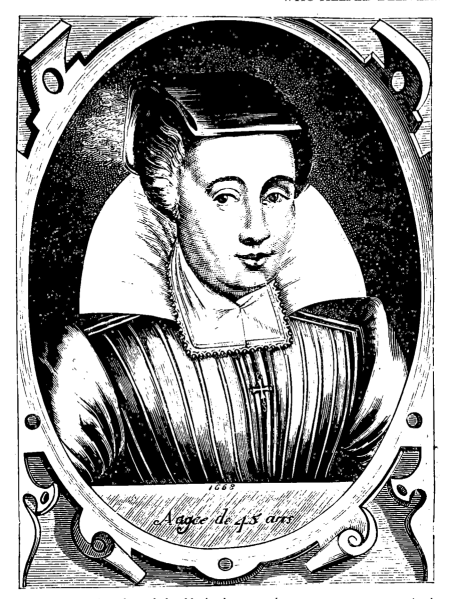

Louise Bourgeois, acknowledged by both men and women as a great expert in the field of midwifery.

Louise Bourgeois also noted the danger of infection for the parturient woman, and her account is probably the first reported description of cross-infection by a midwife.

The example set by Louise and others like her was important because it demonstrated that women could be at least as efficient, if not more

65

competent than the man midwife or doctor. However, the majority of
midwives operated in the rural areas and were very different from the
urban trained midwife. Most 'traditional' midwives were old women who
had no other means of support, and who turned to midwifery out of sheer
necessity. Although in some country areas the office of midwife was one
of prestige and was elected by the local community,[13] in many others it
conferred no status whatever and simply represented a cheap alternative
to the doctor or trained midwife. The staff of a midwifery school set up in
Calau in the eighteenth century claimed that the peasants themselves
regarded midwifery as suited only to women who 'possessed no further
feeling for honour or shame' and became midwives only to confess to the
world their desperation at not making a livelihood in a more honourable
way.[14]

The work of the midwife was so hard and so badly paid that few wanted
it. Not only did the granny midwife often have to turn out at all times of
the day and night, but she might also have

> to stay up all night with her until the infant was baptised, to wash out
> the diapers and swaddling clothes, to invite the guests to the
> baptismal feast, and to change the infant daily until the mother's
> churching, at least three weeks.[15]

Unlike the urban or trained midwives, these women did not regard their
work as a profession, and had no knowledge of anatomy. Most did not
practise full time, and most of their knowledge came from trial and error
and adhering to tradition. At best they had the patience to trust in nature
and let it take its course, but at worst they would intervene constantly,
anxious to prove their worth, or placed under extreme pressure of time
because of another delivery in the community.

> It's country fair time, and a number of old women are hanging
> around the merchants' stands, filling their baskets with laxative
> pills, uterus drops, easy labour drops, tranquillisers and so forth.
> Who are they? Midwives, doing doctor duty . . . [when called to
> attend a labour]. They carry on their backs a heavy birthing stool,
> which also doubles as a potty chair . . . If the cervix is even slightly
> dilated the mother has to climb onto the chair immediately. [They
> smear the vagina] with stinking oils, labour creams, marjoram,
> saffron and brandy, one after the other . . .[16]

There are many recorded instances of midwives puncturing the sac of
amniotic fluid in an effort to speed up events, ignoring the dangers to the
baby. Similarly, it was reported of midwives:

> They stick their hands continuously into the vagina. They stretch it,
> pull it, and manipulate it as though it had a strong, stubborn will of
> its own. They sigh and groan so expressively that one would despair
> of ever seeing the infant actually born.[17]

Because of fears that the uterus would close and prevent delivery of the placenta, there were often attempts to extract it before it was ready. The midwife would pull on the umbilical cord, and if part of the placenta was left behind, she might reach in with her hand to try and locate it. In addition to the possibility of infection, such action could also cause haemorrhage or inversion of the uterus.

That such practices were common is borne out by the number of legal ordinances designed to set limits on the activities of midwives. In 1737, for example, the city of Kaufbeuren in Germany forbade midwives to keep one fingernail long in order to rupture the waters.[18] Some decrees limited manual intervention to supporting the perineum; others forbade midwives from placing women on birthing stools before the waters had broken, and further orders forbade them from pressing back the coccyx to allow the baby to pass.[19]

During the eighteenth century when, particularly in Europe, efforts were being made to ensure that midwives were properly trained, the peasant reliance on time-honoured routine was so great that many resisted the new ways. In 1775 one doctor wrote that rural midwives were

> ... guided by a murderous routine, denuded of any understanding and ridden with prejudices as hurtful as they are numerous. Their lackings are grave, even fatal, for almost all of them begin to practise the art of midwifery without knowing anything, without having learned anything.[20]

Despite the continued use of the granny midwife, even when a trained midwife was available, and despite the reluctance of the granny midwife to learn new ways, proper training slowly made headway, with many midwifery schools being established in Germany and in France in the late eighteenth century. The proper training of midwives was vital for the reduction of the mortality rate, but it also helped to safeguard the position of the female midwife as she came under increasing pressure from the man midwife in the late eighteenth and nineteenth centuries. In Britain, and in America where such training did not exist, the threat from men came earlier.

MIDWIFERY IN BRITAIN

The seventeenth century

In Britain, as in Europe, the Church had imposed regulations on the midwife. In Britain, though, control of the midwife remained in the hands of the Church and did not pass to municipal authorities. Midwives continued to be required to apply to Bishops' courts for a licence. In addition, they had to have character witnesses and be able to present 'six honest matrons' to vouch for safe deliveries. There was, though, little concern shown for technical competence, and there were no exams such as those conducted in Europe. Women who practised without a licence ran the risk of being prohibited or even excommunicated if caught, but the cost of such a licence excluded many, particularly among the rural poor, and most of these midwives continued to practise regardless of the consequences.

Yet because every woman who could conceive was likely to give birth at least once, the midwife was an integral part of society whatever her training or lack of it. In addition to attending birth, she was often called upon to perform other duties, such as searching a woman for proof of adultery or the devil's marks — a sure sign of witchcraft — or examining a woman trying to escape punishment on the grounds of pregnancy.

Midwifery could be a lucrative trade, and attendance at a royal birth brought particularly handsome rewards. Alice Dennis, who attended Anne of Denmark, wife of James I, was paid £100 on two occasions.[1] Later in the seventeenth century Madame Peronne, a French midwife who attended Henrietta Maria, was given £1,000 for successfully delivering the future Charles II.[2] At the bottom of the scale, attendance at a birth at the beginning of the century was rewarded by little more than a shilling or two. In addition to the payment for delivery, though, there were often payments made by godparents. Samuel Pepys, the diarist, paid ten shillings to the midwife on the birth of his godchild.[3]

Midwives regarded themselves as the rightful attendants of birth, 'knowing the cases of women better than any other'.[5] The Holy Scriptures were cited in support, for they 'hath recorded Midwives to the perpetual honour of the female Sex, there being not so much one word concerning Men-midwives mentioned there'.[5]

The man midwife's activities, indeed, were mainly confined to birth where surgery was the only solution, but in the early seventeenth century an instrument was invented which for the first time could extract the child alive where manual skills were not enough. This instrument, forceps, was the brainchild of the Chamberlen brothers — who rather confusingly were both called Peter. When word of their invention spread they were employed at Court, and soon became firm favourites. As it became known that the Chamberlens could shorten labour, many women of standing wanted to be delivered by them and, much to their discredit, the Chamberlens went to great lengths to guard their secret and further the mystique surrounding it. They would arrive at a confinement with a huge wooden box carved in gilt; two people needed to carry it in, the patient was blindfolded and the midwife was ushered out. Then to the sound of ringing bells and the slapping of wooden sticks so that the noise of metal blades was disguised, they would set to work. So successful were they at concealing the design of their instruments that it remained a family secret for nearly a hundred years.

Ironically, since the Chamberlen forceps were in the long run to play a major part in the displacement of the midwife, it was they who first put forward a scheme for the proper training of midwives. They wanted to instruct midwives themselves and bring midwifery into line with standards on the Continent. The plan was rejected by the College of Physicians and by the London midwives, who regarded it as a ploy by the Chamberlens to line their own pockets, but was later revived by Peter Chamberlen III. In a pamphlet entitled 'A Crie of Women and Children echoed forth in the compassion of Peter Chamberlen', he blamed the ignorance of midwives on the physicians and the Church. His plan, too, was rejected.

The midwives who opposed the Chamberlen schemes rested their case on the importance of experience:

> . . . it must be continual practise in this kind that will bring experience, and those women that desire to learn must be present at the delivery of many women and see the work and behaviour of such as be skilful midwives who will shew and direct them and resolve their doubt.[6]

They also added that they possessed books in English on anatomy and, 'most of them being able to read', they believed they would benefit more from them than from Dr Chamberlen's proposed lectures on anatomy. Such midwives were, though, a minority and in 1670 the man midwife Percival Willughby wrote:

> I have been with some that could not read, with several that could not write, and with many that understood very little practice, and for such as these be, it would do no good to speak to them of anatomising the womb.[7]

Until proper training facilities on a par with those offered by the Hôtel Dieu were available, there was little chance of midwifery improving, but in 1671 a landmark was established with the publication of the first text book written by an English midwife. Jane Sharp poked fun at men midwives for their pretentious use of Greek and Latin names. 'It is not hard words that perform the work,' she wrote, 'as if none understood the Art of midwifery that cannot understand Greek.'[8] She believed in sustaining a woman's strength during labour and keeping her warm afterwards. She was opposed to attempts to speed up labour, warned of the difficulty of breech presentation and was aware of the danger of haemorrhage while removing the placenta. However, her book is also riddled with superstitious beliefs.

The last part of the seventeenth century saw one more attempt to revive the Chamberlen scheme, and to ensure that Britain could produce

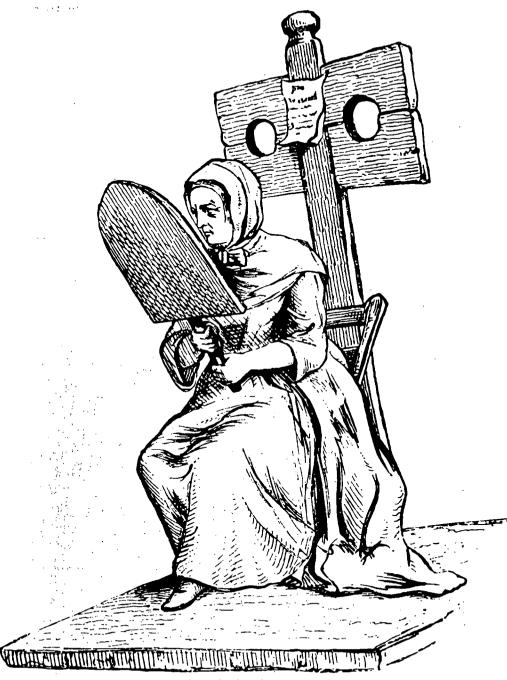

Elizabeth Cellier, an English midwife who suggested setting up a midwives' college. She had a somewhat chequered career, which included a spell in the stocks.

midwives on a par with those on the Continent. It was the brainchild of a Catholic midwife called Elizabeth Cellier but, like the schemes before it, it foundered. The lack of an organised body for midwives was to make them particularly vulnerable in the next century.

At the end of the seventeenth century, the role of the man midwife was still restricted to the small percentage of the population which could afford his fees, or to emergencies, but his supposedly superior education, and most importantly, his instruments, were to make him a very real threat.

The eighteenth century — the rise of the man midwife

Much of the growth in popularity of the man midwife has been attributed to fashion. The decision by Louis XIV of France to employ a court physician, Boucher, to deliver his favourite mistress, Louise de la Valliere in 1663, and again a man, Jules Clement, to deliver the Dauphine in 1682, was highly influential. French courtiers were quick to emulate the king and the fad of employing an 'accoucheur' soon spread.

> The few physicians who were known to be qualified in this art soon found themselves besieged by royalty and the well-to-do, and

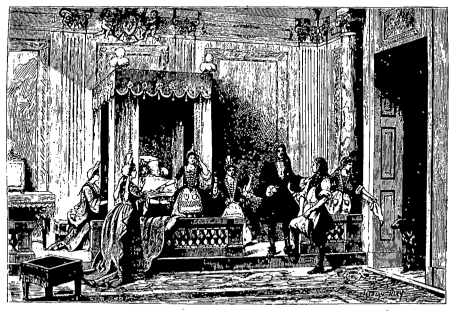

The Dauphine Anne-Victoire being delivered by Jules Clement in 1682. The unfortunate sheep coming through the door was flayed alive and its fleece wrapped round the Dauphine, a popular remedy following a difficult birth. The poor Dauphine was then sealed in her room without light for nine days.

amazed at this sudden turn in their fortunes, they promptly limited their practice to obstetrics.[9]

The fortunes of fashion apart, real progress was being made in establishing birth as a medical science. The groundwork of this 'new midwifery', pioneered by men like Smellie, Fielding Ould and William Hunter, was to make obstetrics a recognised branch of medicine.

The most important credentials of the man midwife were his instruments, in particular the forceps. The design of the forceps used by the Chamberlens was not made public until 1733, although other designs had been available to all male — and almost no female — practitioners of midwifery for some time before then.

Why the forceps were rarely used by midwives is difficult to understand since they played such an important part in wresting control of the birth process from the midwife. Perhaps because they appeared late in the history of the midwife, they never really became part of the skilled woman's tradition. Although there was no legal prohibition, earlier restrictions on the use of the instruments by the midwife may also have had an effect. Possibly instruments were already too closely associated with the destruction of the fetus.

Elizabeth Nihell, a midwife who had trained at the Hotel Dieu school for midwives, was an outspoken enemy of the man midwife in the eighteenth century. She noted that:

> A few, and a very few indeed of the midwives, dazzled with that vogue into which the instruments brought the men ... attempted to employ them, and though certainly they could handle them at least as dextrously as men, they soon discovered that they were at once insignificant and dangerous substitutes to their own hands, with which they were sure of conducting their operations both more safely, more effectually and with less pain to the patient.[10]

The degree of physical strength needed to implement the forceps and the cost of purchasing them may similarly have acted as deterrents. Whatever the reasons, most midwives left forceps to doctors, and many felt that more women died at the hands of the man midwife with his instruments than at the hands of even the most ignorant female midwife. Even William Hunter, a leading exponent of midwifery, said of the forceps that 'where they save one they murder twenty'.[11]

By the middle of the eighteenth century the issue of forceps was one of bitter dispute. In 1758 Elizabeth Nihell published her 400-page polemic, *A Treatise on the Art of Midwifery*, reinforcing the view that men misused instruments. She claimed that too often forceps were used to speed up delivery unnecessarily to impress the family, thus permitting men to ask for a higher fee. This widespread abuse left many children with disabilities and gave rise to the loss of more rather then fewer

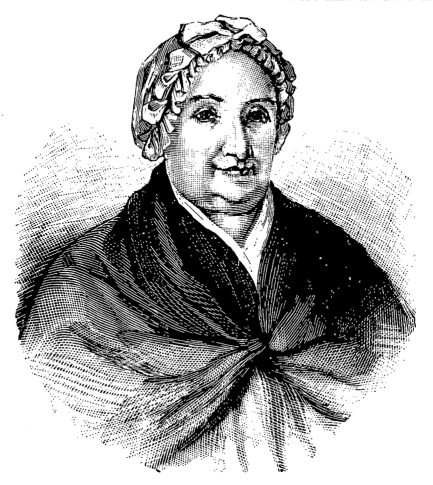

Elizabeth Nihell, one of the most stalwart opponents of the man midwife.

children. Referring to the midwife-teacher William Smellie's pupils, she described them as

> . . . that multitude of disciples . . . those self-constituted man-midwives made out of broken barbers, tailors, or even pork butchers, for I know one myself of this last trade who, having passed half his life in stuffing sausage, is turned out intrepid physician and man-midwife.[12]

Along with many other midwives she claimed that men midwives deliberately mistaught their pupils so that they would be called in to correct their errors. The existence of men midwives also threatened an important area of women's employment.

On the whole, educated physicians agreed with the argument that nature should be sufficient and they advocated non-interference. In 1724 Dr John Maubray in *The Female Physician* wrote:

> However I know, some Chirurgeon-Practitioners are too much acquainted with the Use of *INSTRUMENTS*, to lay them aside; no, they do not (it may be) think themselves in their *Duty*, or proper *Office*, if they have not their cruel Accoutrements in Hand. And what is most unaccountable and unbecoming a Christian is that, when they have perhaps wounded the *MOTHER*, kill'd the *INFANT*, and with violent *Torture* and inexpressible *Pain*, drawn it out by Piece-meal, they think no reward sufficient for such an extraordinary piece of mangled work.[13]

Opposition to men midwives was not only founded on their use or misuse of instruments. Many women still disliked the idea of being attended by a man, and many men, too, regarded it as unseemly to have a man midwife in attendance.

There was also the fear that the man midwife would weaken wifely fidelity. Through their contact with these men, it was argued, women would be more likely to accept other men's advances, and the man midwife himself would have to be superhuman to resist the temptations he was afforded. One writer in 1764 showed the man midwife as travelling from one conquest to another 'like the Emperor of Morocco, or the Bashaw of Tangier, going to his Seraglio'.[14] Later in the century another opponent of male midwifery branded men midwives as the worst evils inflicted on women, together with French dances, novels and boarding schools.[15]

In spite of opposition, the popularity of men midwives grew. Gradually they began to take the better-paid work off the women, and to be paid higher for the same work. Little was done to protect the position of the female midwife. As the power of the Church waned, the system of episcopal licensing became increasingly ineffective, and by the end of the century its breakdown was all but complete. Some areas had already attempted to institute new systems. In Edinburgh the Incorporation of Surgeons, appalled by the frequency of obstetric disasters, asked the Town Council for some form of training to be instigated. In response the Council set up a system of municipal licensing on Continental lines, and in 1726 appointed Joseph Gibson to the first chair of Midwifery anywhere in the world. Glasgow in 1740 instituted a similar system of examination and licensing for midwives of the city and its outskirts.

In Britain, however, no training comparable to that of the Hotel Dieu in France was available. In 1739 Sir Richard Manningham, a leading man midwife, did establish two wards in London to serve as a 'charitable infirmary' for the relief of poor married women in Westminster, and both male and female students were accepted for instruction. Manningham hoped that soon Parliament would take it upon itself to establish a national hospital to serve all lying-in women: it was to be 200 years before his ideal was realised.

Manningham's example was followed in some places, however, and lying-in wards were set up in the Middlesex Hospital in 1747 and the British and City of London lying-in hospitals in 1749 and 1750. In 1752 the Jermyn Street Hospital (known as the General Lying-in Hospital) was founded, and this later became the Queen's Hospital and finally Queen Charlotte's. In 1765 the Westminster New Lying-in Hospital was founded.

In Ireland, men were also becoming involved with birth. Benjamin Mosse, a licentiate in midwifery of the King's and Queen's College of Physicians, had been horrified to discover the terrible conditions of squalor in which some of his Dublin patients lived. Founding a committee with some friends, he bought a house for the poor which in 1745 became the Hospital for Poor Lying-in Women. When it became clear that its twelve beds were grossly insufficient, the site of the Dublin Rotunda was bought in 1748 to furnish 150 beds.

In Scotland there were similar developments. In 1756 Thomas Young, then the Professor of Midwifery in Edinburgh, persuaded the Royal Infirmary to let him use an attic room for four lying-in women. The room was replaced in 1793 when Alexander Hamilton opened the Edinburgh General Lying-in Hospital, all costs being borne by him and his son, James, who was Professor of Midwifery after his father. In Glasgow, James Towers established a small lying-in institution at his own expense, and offered clinical instruction in midwifery at a time when the subject was not compulsory in the medical curriculum. In Aberdeen, wards for poor lying-in women were also set up.

Most of these hospitals were very small. They were run by male governors, and the matron in charge would be subordinate to the medical officers. They did provide midwives with instruction but, importantly, they were also providing men with a ready source of clinical material.

In London and other major towns, further skilled assistance was offered by the 'out-door charities',[16] similar to modern outpatient schemes. The larger charities sometimes trained midwives free. In return for training, the midwives agreed to work for the charity at a low fee for a period of time. Because these midwives were free to take on private practice as well, they had the advantage of serving poor and rich clients at the same time. Outdoor charities did not provide food or lodging, so they were cheaper than hospitals for the parturient woman. They were also safer since patients were not subjected to the epidemics of puerperal fever which bedevilled hospitals.

The second half of the century saw voluntary training organisations multiply yet none of the training facilities compared with those which were set up in Europe in the eighteenth century. Until proper provision of training for midwives, the old working class woman who attended the poor would continue to connive in sexual intrigues, perform abortions, run lying-in homes for prostitutes and shelter unwanted babies. So the 'old crone' image of the midwife was perpetuated, while better educated women were discouraged from midwifery because of the image of the profession and lack of financial reward. The immediate beneficiary of all this was the man midwife, and during the nineteenth century male practice in midwifery became more general in England than anywhere else in Europe.

The nineteenth century and the fight for regulation

The man midwife

By the beginning of the nineteenth century it was clear that regulation of midwifery practice was essential to ensure the survival of the midwife. Recognition of the professional standing of the man midwife too was slow in coming. Men midwives were for long regarded as 'mongrel physicians', forced to invade the province of women because they could not succeed in orthodox medicine. Such a view had both professional and social consequences. At the beginning of the century, for example, the wife of James Hamilton, Professor of Midwifery at Edinburgh, found herself cold-shouldered at a charity ball because of her husband's profession.[17]

When the nineteenth century opened, there was no formal teaching of midwifery in the medical schools (apart from Edinburgh), and none of the universities or diploma-granting bodies included midwifery among the subjects of its final examination. In the late eighteenth century the College of Physicians had honoured a few distinguished men midwives, conferring on them a licence of midwifery, but in 1804 they followed the lead taken by the College of Surgeons and instituted a bye-law prohibiting men midwives from election to their fellowship.[18]

The first organised move to improve the standards of midwifery was made in 1813, when the Society of Apothecaries tried to persuade Parliament to pass legislation to regulate the medical profession and suppress unqualified practice. They protested against the unsatisfactory state of midwifery and wanted legislation passed for the education and control of midwives. Their proposals were introduced into the House as a Bill but the Commons Committee would not allow any mention of women midwives, and the matter was dropped. Eventually one tiny step was made when the College of Surgeons agreed to demand certificates of attendance at midwifery lectures from candidates who applied for their diploma.

The obstacles encountered in gaining even minor concessions demonstrates the degree of hostility from the medical profession that still existed towards the men midwives. In 1827 Sir Henry Halford, President of the College of Physicians, explained to Sir Robert Peel that it should not 'create surprise' that midwifery, being a manual operation was 'deemed foreign to the habits of Gentlemen of enlarged academical education'.[19] A similar view was taken by Sir Anthony Carlisle, later President of the College of Surgeons. In May 1827, he wrote a letter to *The Times* condemning men midwives and the Obstetrical Society's attempts to 'regularise' such a 'dishonourable vocation'. In 1834 he told a Select Committee of the House of Commons that 'it is an imposture to pretend that a medical man is required at labour'. [20] Like many others he regarded childbirth as a natural process which had been invaded for pecuniary reward. Instead he felt that midwives should be women, preferably wives or relations of surgeons or apothecaries as was common on the Continent.

In 1836 the Act for the Registration of Births, Marriages and Deaths in England and Wales at last made national statistics on maternal mortality available. Dr William Farr, superintendent of the new Registrar-General's office, in his report of 1841, was outspoken in his attacks on the lack of training of midwives. His research revealed that over 3,000 mothers died each year (many in fact of puerperal fever), and he believed that this number would be greatly reduced by proper training in midwifery generally.

Despite Dr Farr's report and many other stories of negligence and harm caused by male and female midwives, the traditional British distrust of any extension of the powers of central government was still strong. The Chemist Registration Act of 1852 merely distinguished between qualified and unqualified practitioners; and in the same way the Medical Act of 1858 which was meant to regulate the medical profession, carried no penalty for unqualified practitioners.

By the middle of the century, however, men midwives had achieved some success in their attempts to improve the teaching of midwifery and to be recognised by the medical profession. Gradually the derisive title man midwife was dropped in favour of the more stately title 'obstetrician', meaning 'to stand before'. This had the advantage of sounding more professional. More importantly, several colleges were permitting midwifery to be included in their curricula, and some even examined in it. The first concessions in this area were made in Scotland, and Ireland was in advance of England too. In London the field was led by University College.

In 1852 the College of Surgeons finally relented and set up a midwifery licence for those who wanted the qualification. Like the College of Physicians, it abandoned the bye-law prohibiting election of midwifery practitioners to its council. The conjoint board examinations, however, did not include obstetricians until as late as 1886.

In 1858 a new Obstetrical Society was formed, aimed at putting obstetrics on an equal footing with other branches of medicine and with membership open to any registered medical practitioner. There was still much to be done with regard to proper training facilities.

Although all London and most provincial medical schools had by now a lecturer in obstetrics, and most schools appointed an obstetrician to the honorary medical staff in the 1850s and 60s, few medical school hospitals allotted beds for training in obstetrics.

Despite the constant urging for students to attend a number of births, lack of accommodation rarely allowed it. In the 1870s in Edinburgh, for example, there were over 1,000 students but only 7,000 births 'of the rank of life that made them suitable to undergraduates'.[21] Even in the 1890s a typical student in a large London hospital would attend only one birth in the week allotted for obstetric rotation. One such student was, moreover

> not permitted to touch the patient. After the child was delivered the patient was taken away, he never saw her or the child again. He and his colleagues asked to be shown the obstetric instruments: the consultant refused, saying their request was 'most irregular'; he sent them to obtain 'special permission', which was refused. [The student] and his friends at the end of the week were certified as having attended the whole number of deliveries that occurred in the hospital during the week. He was thereby qualified in the words of his certificate 'to undertake anything required in obstetrics'.[22]

With so little training in even normal births, doctors had no background information to help them in an abnormal delivery. It was hardly surprising that many young general practitioners were obstetrically incompetent. Yet the numbers of doctors increased by 53 per cent in the thirty years after 1831, rising from 17,300 to 26,500[23] and it was this new breed of obstetrician which was to form a major hurdle to the midwife in her search for recognition.

The midwife

The nineteenth century was, for the most part, the dark age of the midwife. Elizabeth Nihell's warnings about the erosion of job opportunities for women were well founded. Much traditional women's work was being taken over by men, and as a result there was a growing surplus of labour on the market.

In a society so enveloped in prudery that the 'leg' could only be called a 'limb' and the 'limbs' of a pianoforte could be found dressed in trousers,[24]

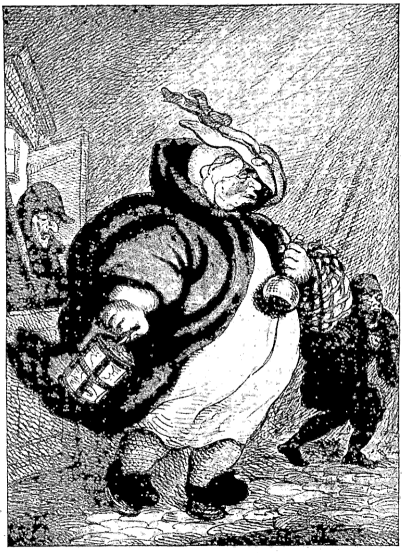

MIDWIFE GOING TO LABOR; A CARICATURE BY ROWLANDSON, 1800

This rotund "Sairey Gamp" has been called to an early-morning case. In one hand she carries her lantern and in the other a bottle of brandy and her luggage. She is mounted on pattens to escape the mud of the streets. A sleepy chimney-sweep with his brushes and bags crouches along beside her.

79

midwifery was no longer regarded as a respectable occupation for a woman. Particulary damaging to the midwife was the belief that women were intellectually and physically inferior to men. It was felt that even if a woman was given the necessary training she would never be able to use obstetric instruments with precision. Increasingly, it was accepted that the use of instruments should be left to men.

Lack of work in other fields, though, led defenders of the midwife to advocate midwifery as a suitable employment for the *single* woman for the first time. Some even suggested that women should study all female diseases so that they would be able to consult other women rather than men. As a writer to the *Examiner* in June 1827 expressed it:

> How many myriads of young and shrinking females . . . have been consumed by diseases which delicacy compelled them to conceal from a man, but which they might readily have submitted to a physician of their sex.[25]

In 1830 the new British Ladies Lying-in Institute was founded with the aim of providing well-trained women not only for the charitable care of the poor but also for private practice. Its midwives were at first instructed by a lady, Mrs C M Beale, but in 1858 a surgeon-accoucheur took over and midwives were once again subordinate to men.

By 1851 the growing number of women in Britain was giving rise to concern. There were now half a million more women than men in the 20-40 age group.[26] Large numbers of single women in the working class could still find employment in domestic, factory or field work — sweated labour generally — and prostitution. The only respectable outlet for the single middle-class woman was still as a governess. The surplus of women had to be accommodated: and the reason that change came about was in large part due to the concerted political action — for the first time — of middle-class women willing and able to devote time to the cause of women. The emergence of women like Florence Nightingale and Elizabeth Fry as figures of national note was a boost to their crusade.

Slowly the legal position of women began to improve. In 1839 the Infant's Custody Act allowed women living apart from their husbands rights to their children. In 1857 the Marriage and Divorce Bill resulted in an Act making divorce easier and giving some protection to women who had been deserted and who could now keep their own earnings. Until 1884, however, women could be imprisoned for denial of conjugal rights, and until 1891 a husband could forcibly prevent his wife from leaving him. It was only towards the end of the century that three Married Women's Property Acts accorded women proper legal rights.

The need to promote employment for women began to concern philanthropic organisations. In 1859 the Society for Promoting Employment of Women set about trying to expand the opportunities for women. A variety of suitable employments were advocated from book-keeping to shoe making. Nursing was also included largely because of the efforts of Florence Nightingale during the Crimean War. Midwifery was not recommended as a suitable employment but Miss Nightingale herself wanted to see the status of the midwife improved. In 1861 she opened an annexe of her hospital in which she hoped to train midwives to work among the rural poor. Unfortunately, her plans were bedevilled by an outbreak of puerperal fever in the hospital, originating from a woman who was delivered while suffering from erysipelas. She was forced to close it down, and no-one else followed the lead she had made.

Women were also attempting around this time to break into the medical profession. Women in America had already made some headway in this field and in 1856 Jessie Meriton White applied to the Royal College of Surgeons and the University of London asking to be admitted to their examination. She was turned down, but in 1856 Elizabeth Garrett Anderson passed the examination of the Society of Apothecaries, demonstrating that women were capable of qualifying for the Register.

In 1864 the Female Medical Society which had formed in 1862, founded the 'Ladies' Medical College'. The society's long-term aim was to force the entry of women into medicine, but their immediate goal was to establish midwifery as a suitable occupation for gentlewomen. They set

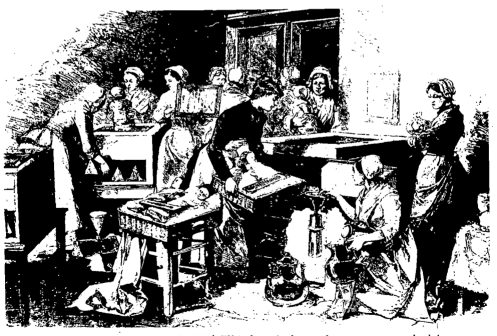

Scene in the Paris Maternité, 1884. This hospital was the successor to the lying-in wards of the Hotel Dieu. It was here that incubators for babies, warmed by kerosone, were first used.

out to supply skilled female practitioners for ladies, and to open up an honourable and lucrative form of employment for educated women. The College soon had twenty women in attendance, the majority of whom were single or widows, hoping to attend gentlewomen as well as the poor. Apart from midwifery, pupils had also to have an understanding of the diseases peculiar to women and children.

The improved training of these midwives may have raised the status of the midwife in some eyes, but it did nothing to solve the problem of the great number of totally uninstructed midwives in the rest of the country. Many of these combined midwifery with laying out the dead or some other menial work in order to make a living.

In 1866 Dr William Farr suggested to the Obstetrical Society that there should be an investigation into the causes of infant mortality. The report revealed that midwives still attended 70 per cent of all births in England and Wales[27] and that most had no instruction, were grossly ignorant and often incompetent. In response to that report and in an attempt to lower the infant mortality rate of 160 per 1,000 live births, the Obstetrical Society proposed the registration of still births and the prohibition of all unqualified midwives, male and female. In 1872 it set up its own examining board and a diploma. In Scotland, too, examinations were set and certificates awarded.

The reputation of the midwife was at a particularly low ebb at this time. In 1870 Mrs Waters, a 'baby farmer' was put on trial, and then hanged for the murder of one of the children in her care. A midwife, Mrs Hall, was also involved. She ran a private lying-in home in which she provided refuge for women having illegitimate babies. The babies were passed on to Mrs Waters, who subjected them to a regime of neglect, starvation and slow poisoning.[28] The case focused public attention once more on the midwife issue.

By the 1870s the opposing sides were drawn up in a struggle that was to last until the end of the century. Many members of the Women's Rights movements who saw that the prospects for women were opening up, feared that midwife regulation which placed them under a rival body would restrict female employment rather than secure it. Many midwives feared a registration system that linked them to attendance at normal births only. And the medical profession increasingly urged registration that would keep midwives subordinate.

In 1874 the Female Medical Society closed. Its demise marked the end of the hopes of those like Florence Nightingale, that Britain could produce midwives of the scientific distinction of some European midwives. From now on women seeking a recognised qualification in midwifery on an equal basis with men had to struggle to be admitted to the Medical Register as medical practitioners.

Elizabeth Garrett Anderson had got on the Medical Register by passing the exams of the Society of Apothecaries. That particular loophole was then closed, and it seemed impossible once more for a woman to become a doctor. On the one hand she was barred from getting the necessary clinical training in hospitals and dissecting rooms; on the other she was forbidden by Act of Parliament from practising without them. However, Sophia Jex Blake and her Edinburgh colleagues refused to accept defeat. In 1875 she founded the London School of Medicine for Women and by 1878 women were able to gain clinical instruction at the Royal Free Hospital.

The acceptance of women as doctors was a spectacular victory. For the first time the way was clear for midwife registration to be dealt with as a separate issue. However, there were still problems — notably the form registration should take. Many women feared that the scheme put forward by the Obstetrical Society would limit women's opportunities and place them under a rival organisation. The medical profession, conversely, did not want midwives usurping the general practitioner who was increasingly finding midwifery a lucrative sideline.

About the only point on which all proponents of registration agreed was that untrained, unsupervised midwives did much harm — and it is by no means certain that this assumption was correct. No mortality figures for midwifery as a whole existed and, on the contrary, statistics for the practice of midwives in a number of 'out-door' charities showed a rate of less than half the 5 deaths per 1,000 estimated by Dr Farr for the nation as a whole. Farr himself pointed out that if many midwives fell below this high standard so too did many medical men.[29] The highest death rates were in the hospitals into which the poor were herded, risking exposure to puerperal fever and greater danger than if they had delivered at home.[30] Naturally there were obstetricians who were reluctant to accept the theory that poor women living in the slums and attended by imperfectly educated midwives were less at risk from infection than well-to-do patients attended by skilled obstetricians.

Attempts to find common ground enough to push through registration enactment went on. In 1881 the Matron's Aid or Trained Midwives' Registration Society was founded, renamed in 1889 the Midwives' Institute. The leaders of the new society realised that they needed the help of leading obstetricians if a midwives' Bill was ever to be passed. Accordingly they accepted that their midwives, while being competent to cope with normal labour, would be prepared to send for a doctor when complications arose. Haunted by the Sairey Gamp image of the drunken midwife in Dickens' *Martin Chuzzlewit*, they were particularly careful in their choice of members. Appealing directly to the evangelical religious ethos which was the driving force for so much philanthropy, they laid down strict rules of conduct. There must be no drinking or discussion of cases, and members should try to have a moral influence on the whole family, encouraging mothers to regard their children as gifts from God.

Such sentiments may have been laudable, but they had little meaning for the traditional midwife who had witnessed so often the debilitating effect of bearing many children. Many such midwives were valued because of their willingness to help mothers already overburdened with children by arranging for the early demise of their newest arrival. Indeed this 'churchyard luck' was often an important credential for a midwife in the eyes of her clientele.[31]

The first legislative measure for midwives was introduced into the House of Commons in 1890, and it soon became clear that the Bill would not be plain sailing. The most important element in the opposition to the Bill was the body of less affluent medical practitioners who feared that a Bill for midwives would threaten their livelihoods and rob them of a large part of their income.

A number of Bills introduced between 1890 and 1897 went the way of the first one. By that time the British Medical Association was under increasing pressure to include more severe restrictions on midwives. Childbirth which had at the beginning of the nineteenth century been regarded as a natural process needing no medical intervention was now viewed as a perpetual hazard requiring medical assistance.

By 1900, moreover, the social climate had begun to change following the defeats of the Boer War (1899-1901). Many had been shocked by the generally poor health of the fighting men of the nation, and it was now considered more acceptable that medical attendance on poor childbearing women should be financed from the public purse.

The midwife issue was further highlighted in 1901 because of the wide publicity surrounding two childbirth fatalities. In the first case, in Kent, the husband had applied to three doctors when complications had arisen; all had refused to attend because they did not want to follow a midwife. In the second case, in Stepney, as a consequence of which an elderly midwife was imprisoned for manslaughter, the husband had called a doctor. The doctor had, however, excused himself because he might be charged with 'covering' unqualified practice by the General Medical Council. The incidents served to expose the danger of doctors refusing to attend cases in which a midwife had been in charge. In some areas trained midwives in private practice or in maternal charities were being forced to leave the district because they did not want the responsibility for attending abnormal cases on their own.

The year 1902 was to see the end of twelve years of controversy. Finally a Midwives' Act went on the Statute Book. It was of necessity a compromise, but it was also a humiliation for bodies like the General Medical Council and the British Medical Association. It was a real victory for women's organisations, parliament and the government, and for the selfless and unwearied service of many medical men too. The Act made provision for state registration instead of annual licensing, and midwives had to inform local authorities of their intent to practise. Unqualified midwives were to be prohibited — but not until 1910, which allowed a period in which they could obtain qualifications.

The intense medical opposition had meant that a Bill could be passed only with a vast amount of public support; and this had been achieved. Yet the midwife remained uniquely disadvantaged compared with other professions, for she was subject to local authority supervision and regulated by a rival profession. It would not have been possible, though, to sustain public opinion in favour of midwife registration indefinitely. Although the Act was repressive in some aspects, it at least conferred compensatory status and halted the decline of the midwife. Without the Act, pressure from medical practitioners would probably have led to the disappearance of the midwife. While obstetric care to this day remains male dominated, the Act defended a traditional female occupation and the right of women to be attended by women in childbirth.

The story in America was a different one.

MIDWIFERY IN AMERICA

Despite the long struggle for regulation, the 1902 Midwives' Act assured the British midwife's place at birth. Her American counterpart enjoyed no such recognition. During the nineteenth century she was displaced in the middle-class home by the doctor, surviving only in the poorest sections of society, among the ethnic immigrants and the poor blacks. Why was the outcome so different?

The colonial midwives of seventeenth-century America came from Britain and brought with them their practices. Birth, as elsewhere, was the exclusive province of women. Expectant mothers relied on the skills of the midwife should anything go wrong. Midwives did not formally train for their work, and had neither an organised guild to license themselves nor a formal apprenticeship. In some colonies a system of civil licensing was instituted. Despite the lack of organisation, though, the colonial midwife seems to have been accorded a high degree of respect and responsibility. The colonists needed children in order to prosper, and malpractices by the midwife were unlikely to have been tolerated. In this new society, moreover, a midwife

> performed her work within a culture that was also changing, so that
> the experiences and expectations of women about birth were not
> always the same.[1]

Some idea of the life of the midwife can be gleaned from the diary of Mrs

Martha Moore Ballard, who practised after the Revolution of 1776, from 1778 to 1812. She was not a trained midwife, but she worked for 34 years and delivered 996 women, recording only four maternal deaths.[2] Although she mentions instances of having to remove an obstruction or extract a placenta by hand, her role seems more commonly to have been to offer reassurance.

The performance of midwives in colonial America seems to have been good; there are no recorded epidemics of puerperal fever caused by midwives, and a medical historian of Virginia has calculated that even the illiterate black midwives in Virginia spread less infection than doctors until the end of the nineteenth century.[3]

It is possible that midwives simply had less need to intervene to help exhausted and unhealthy women than their European counterparts. The colonists had a dependable food supply, and were largely free of the unsanitary effects of urban congestion. They did not suffer from the crises of crop failure, famine or epidemics that in some instances destroyed a third of the population of English and French towns and weakened the survivors. Even in American towns the death rates were between 66 to 80 per cent of the death rate in comparable towns in England and France.[4] In the Southern colonies women's health was probably poorer for environmental and nutritional reasons. Many white women employed wet nurses for their babies and therefore tended to become pregnant again more quickly. Multiparity took its toll of their health.

As in Europe, childbirth was, however, still approached with dread, possibly more because of the cultural emphasis on birth as potential death than because of high rates of mortality. Birth was seen as a direct expression of God's will or the power of the devil. The abnormal child was an indication of the spiritual status of the parents. Because of her association with birth the midwife was often viewed with suspicion and even charged with witchcraft. In fact the first person executed in the Massachusetts Bay colony was Margaret Jones, a midwife convicted of witchcraft.[5]

The Puritan authorities' effectiveness in eliminating the magical practices commonly associated with birth meant that the labouring woman could only call on God's mercy and was denied the ancient forms of comfort derived from superstitious beliefs. The limits this imposed on the midwife are important because they may have weakened her position. Whereas in Britain and Europe the superstitions surrounding birth satisfied women and kept doctors away, in America they simply did not exist.[6] In addition there was another factor:

> ... historians have said that Protestantism bred a cultural acceptance
> of new science and a particular willingness to intervene technically
> in nature. Many American women, whether urban or rural were

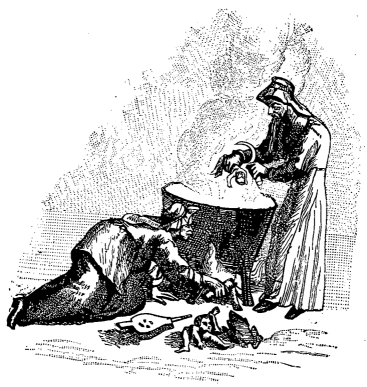

A newborn baby being sacrificed. There are many incidents of midwives being accused of conniving with the devil and the Puritans were particularly vigilant in stamping out magic and superstitious practices in the birth process. (J Sprenger and H Institoris, Malleus Maleficarum.*)*

more ready than the majority of English women to look positively on the doctor's new knowledge and technical skills. Doctors therefore inherited a cultural process that had demystified birth and rationalised it before doctors appeared.[7]

Certainly the better health of American women probably made childbearing a regular process that did not need magic. When difficulties arose it was the fault of nature, to be corrected by manipulating nature with instrumental skill; as a consequence women were more willing to give doctors medical control over birth.

Medicine in America was free of the rivalries between different medical branches that persisted in Europe. Because there were no hospitals or colleges, aspiring doctors were forced to go to Britain or Europe to train. In the period following 1750 they returned armed with new skills — particularly in the field of obstetrics — and they used this knowledge to establish their professional status. If a doctor could satisfy a woman in childbirth, there was every chance he would be called in to deal with the multitude of other ailments that occurred within a family.

At first this posed no threat to the midwife. The view of leading doctors was that in normal cases nature would be adequate and intervention in the birth process unnecessary. As there was also a lack of trained doctors, from 1750 to 1810 midwifery was a shared enterprise. Midwives attended normal births and doctors were called in to attend any complications. A course for midwives was set up in New York in 1799 and another on anatomy and midwifery in Philadelphia. Few women attended but many men did and were trained as men midwives.[8] A scheme was initiated by Dr Thomas Ewell of Washington DC in 1817 to set up a school for midwives attached to a hospital, but when he could not obtain federal funding the project languished.[9] In the United States, unlike in Europe, the government supplied no medical education for midwives, and women alone could not afford to support such a school.

Gradually the plans for a shared midwifery crumbled. The tradition of self help in America was, and remained, strong. Midwives already in practice did not want to be organised, and because there had never been an organised medical profession midwives did not share the European-trained doctors' interest in a shared midwifery enterprise.

Whatever their reasons, the midwives' refusal to be organised was to make them very vulnerable. In the years after 1810 the practice of midwifery in American towns became subject to the same unregulated open-market competition as that which existed in Britain. Men and women of various degrees of training and experience jostled with each other to attend the birth. Even among qualified medical practitioners there was considerable divergence. Medical students began to go to new American colleges to train, and in these colleges midwifery was the first medical speciality, with precedence over surgery because of midwifery's importance as an entrée to medical practice.

Formal qualifications were, of course, no substitute for experience, and one graduate described his terror on being faced with his first delivery:

> I was left alone with a poor Irish woman and one crony, to deliver her child . . . and I thought it necessary to call before me every circumstance I had learned from books — I must examine, and I did — but whether it was head or breech, hand or foot, man or monkey, that was defended from my uninstructed finger by the distended membranes, I was as uncomfortably ignorant, with all my learning, as the foetus itself that was making all this fuss.[10]

The greater number of doctors, furthermore, were poorly educated men who had spent a few months at a proprietary medical school (profit-making concerns owned by local doctors who also taught there), where they gained no practical clinical experience. Writing in 1818, Dr John

Stearns, President of the New York Medical Society, said:

> With a few honourable exceptions in each city, the practitioners are
> ignorant, degraded and contemptible.[11]

Throughout the nineteenth century doctors continued to obtain diplomas
with as little as four months attendance at a school which often had no
laboratories, no dissections and no clinical training.

The poor standards of medical training turned many people to the
unorthodox — Samuel Thomson and his Botanical system of cure based
on roots and herbs, Samuel Hahnemann's homoeopathy where tiny
doses of drugs were applied to help the body recover from disease, or
hydrotherapy, which involved drinking mineral water and taking cold
baths (believed to be particularly efficacious in preventing pain in birth).
The unorthodox sects were many, and the wide variety of choice became a
matter of increasing concern for doctors. Even though educated doctors
had little to offer until the development of bacteriology, they firmly
believed that their training needed some protection. Early licensing laws
were ineffective, and in 1848 the American Medical Association was
formed. It was not, however, until the end of the century that licensing
laws were re-established.

During the nineteenth century the change in cultural attitudes about
the proper place and activity of women in society was another factor in
ensuring the decline of the midwife. It became increasingly unthinkable
that women could be confronted with the facts of medicine or allowed to
mix in a training situation. An anonymous pamphlet published in 1820
represents a complete reversal of the centuries-old argument that only
women should attend birth:

> They have not that power of action, or that active power of mind,
> which is essential to the practice of a surgeon. They have less power
> of restraining and governing the natural tendencies to sympathy and
> are more disposed to yield to the expressions of acute sensibility . . .
> where they become the principal agents, the feelings of sympathy
> are too powerful for the cool exercise of judgement.[12]

Popular theories about menstruation bolstered this view. Many doctors
believed that during menstruation a woman's limited bodily energy was
diverted from the brain, rendering her idiotic — and hence incompetent.
Midwifery training, it was thought, would be an affront to a woman's
modesty and morality. In the dissecting rooms she would taint her moral
character and be, literally, unsexed, subjecting herself to physical exertion
and nervous excitement that would damage her female organs and render
her unable to fulfil her true role as wife and mother. One doctor, Charles
Meigs, in a 'Lecture on the Distinctive Characteristics of the Female'
published in 1847 declaimed that 'She has a head almost too small for

intellect and just big enough for love'.[13] In such a climate of opinion, and lacking any organisation, midwives proved easy targets for the male-dominated medical profession. Rightly or wrongly, most middle and upper-class women came to believe that doctors afforded more safety and respectability.

Not all women, however, accepted the popular notions on the role of women. In 1847 Harriet K Hunt applied to Harvard Medical School. She was turned down. In 1850 she tried again, was admitted to the faculty, but had to withdraw because of objections from the students. In the same year Elizabeth Blackwell was accepted by Geneva Medical School in New York. She graduated at the top of her class, but had to go to Paris and to London to obtain clinical experience, for no American hospital would accept her. On her return in 1856 she established the New York Infirmary for Women and Children, to serve the poor and give women the opportunity for clinical experience. In 1864 she opened a medical college in conjunction with the infirmary, and occupied the first chair of hygiene or preventive medicine in America.

Elizabeth Blackwell's success showed that women could enter the medical profession. In particular, she argued that the care of the children, the sick, the wounded and, most importantly, women in childbirth 'has always been far more the special duty of women than men'. However, although she noted the passing of the midwife in America, it was with no great regret. She regarded the old midwife as an 'imperfect institution' that 'will disappear with the progress of society'. Instead she felt that 'the midwife must give place to the physician. Women must therefore become the physicians.'[14]

Special medical schools were founded for the training of women, but even so, the number of women who acquired medical degrees was small, and they were hindered at every turn. Local medical societies barred them from membership and hospitals refused to give them clinical training. Women did found their own institutions, but their practice was limited and tended to be restricted to serving the poor. The development of nursing as a profession for educated women also drew off many suitable candidates.

The demise of the midwife in America was not without its disadvantages. Doctors began to lose the benefit of combined skills which were still available in Europe. In France, for example, doctors were trained clinically alongside student midwives, and hospital midwives actually trained some doctors in normal deliveries. As a result French doctors did not lose touch with a belief in the powers of nature in birth. In America, while many doctors still advocated non-intervention wherever possible, many young doctors had little clinical training, and had to rely on text books and lectures. They were often embarrassed, confused and frightened by the whole birth process. Doctors did not wish to appear

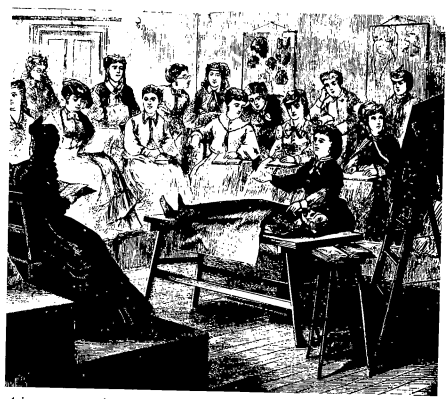

A lecture room of a Homoeopathic Medical School for Women in New York City. (Frank Leslies, Illustrated Weekly Newspaper, *New York, 16 April 1870)*

indifferent, inattentive or useless; they wanted to prove their worth. As a consequence, they tended to intervene more and more. In addition, women began to reinforce this trend because they came to believe that things might go wrong.

The male takeover of control of the birth process during the nineteenth century was far more complete in America than in Europe or even Britain. American society expanded quickly, and a medical profession evolved to serve the new communities. The disappearance of the midwife among the middle classes was not the result of a conspiracy between doctors and husbands. The choice was made by women because they believed doctors would offer them better care; and as the number of educated midwives diminished, women found it harder to find respectable midwives. Women chose men, and eventually there were only men to choose.

By the beginning of the twentieth century, the midwife really only served the ethnic immigrants, the blacks and sections of the poor white communities. In 1906 a New York study was commissioned to examine midwives among the immigrants. It found them hopelessly ignorant, dirty and incompetent, and existing legislation on midwifery practice was tightened accordingly. Birth was moving out of the home and into the hospital, and the natural way of birth began to lose its appeal. A concern for health and a trust in the healing art of the physician went hand in hand. Obstetricians as well as physicians reaped the reward. The midwife, meanwhile, was forgotten.

BIRTH — THE GROWTH OF
THE MEDICAL APPROACH

It is much to be regretted, that there are yet many of the [female] sex,
who are prejudiced in favour of ancient, erroneous opinions and
customs, and thereby exclude themselves from the advantages they
might reap by consulting those who are better acquainted with the
human frame, and have acquired a much greater share of this species
of knowledge . . .

Dr J Grigg, *Advice to the Female Sex in General, Particularly Those
in a State of Pregnancy and Lying In*, 1789, p144.

Nature is perfectly competent to bring without the assistance of
man, a child into this world . . . Assist Nature! Can anything be more
absurd?

P H Chavasse, *Advice to a Wife on the Management of her Own
Health*, 1832 (8th edition 1911), p172.

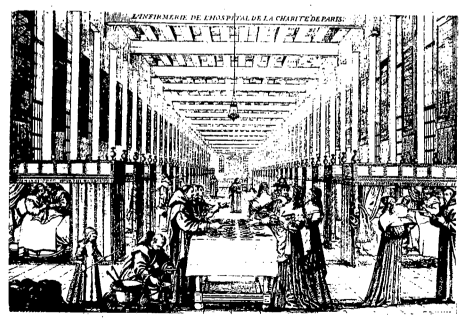

Hospital de la Charité, Paris. (Engraving by Abraham Boss)

MEDICAL PROGRESS

In the past, women approached childbirth with dread more often than joy because they knew from experience that nature was not always orderly and benevolent, that delivery could be painful, destructive and sometimes fatal.

Western women today are physically less burdened than ever before. They have a considerable degree of control over their own fertility, most women's diseases of the past have been eliminated, and birth is

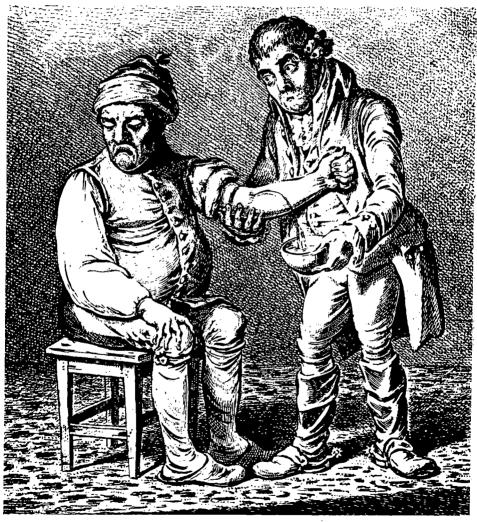

Venesection, or blood letting, was a popular treatment for ill health from the time of the ancient Greeks until the nineteenth century.

95

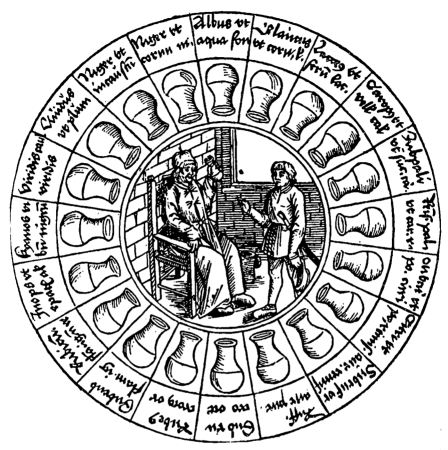

A urine chart. Mediaeval physicians used these to classify the colour of a patient's urine and so diagnose his illness.

altogether a much less risky affair. This has been made possible through the development of medical science, the growth of the profession and the ability to implement scientific and medical discoveries. It has not been a continuous line of progress, however, but a mixture of advance and regression. Too often new discoveries meant that old ways were uncritically discarded. Over the centuries preventive medicine and public hygiene were largely ignored and this brought new problems; but the benefits medical progress brought and the influence of medicine in the field of birth today cannot be ignored.

Early Medicine

It was the Greeks who, borrowing from other civilisations, laid the foundations of western medicine, separating the art of the physician from the cult of the priest, studying disease systematically, and recording the results. Lay practitioners like Hippocrates in the fifth century BC established a system for the practice of the healing arts. Although they believed in nature as the best cure, and in practising interference as little as possible, they were also influenced by the theory of the four humours — blood, phlegm, yellow bile and black bile — of which it was thought the body was made up. Treatments to restore the humours to their correct balance were special foods and bleeding. Bleeding (venesection) remained a common treatment for disease for centuries. The Greeks placed great emphasis on preventive medicine, and on proper diet, sport, and elaborate personal hygiene.

Even after the decline of Greece as a power, Greeks continued to dominate the medical scene. They were to exert an important influence on the Roman practice of medicine, and on their ideas of public health and hygiene. In the field of women's diseases it was two Greeks practising in Rome, Soranus and Rufus, who made the most important contributions: Rufus because of his discovery and naming of various parts of the female anatomy, and Soranus through his book *The Diseases of Women*, which was to be a source book on midwifery for centuries.

Soranus taught a rational midwifery based on knowledge rather than superstition, discouraged brute force, and brought to women in labour more care and kindness and skilled attention than they had yet received. Sadly for women, his advice was lost to the West in the Dark Ages and the early mediaeval period. Instead, the work of another Greek, Galen, dominated the medical scene.

Galen was born in AD 131. His interests were very diverse, but his experimental and anatomical work made valuable contributions. Unfortunately, most of his dissection was done on animals whose anatomy he believed corresponded to that of humans, and thus incorporated many misconceptions. Galen produced a complete system of medicine and provided a mass of detailed and well-organised information. His descriptions of anatomy and physiology were influenced by the theory that all the organs in the body had been produced by a 'Creator' for some definite purpose. These ideas, often distorted, were to have a special appeal to Muslims and Christians, and ensured the survival of his work in the centuries to come. Galen's death in AD 200 was said to have ushered in 'a thousand years of darkness'.[1] Most of the teachings of the Greeks were lost following the Islamic invasion of the West in the 7th century, but the Arabs amassed a huge library of Greek manuscripts which eventually filtered back into western society and these, together with their own contributions, came to form an important part of mediaeval medical knowledge.

The gradual spread of Christianity in the West may have reimposed order on a society which had disintegrated, but it did little to halt

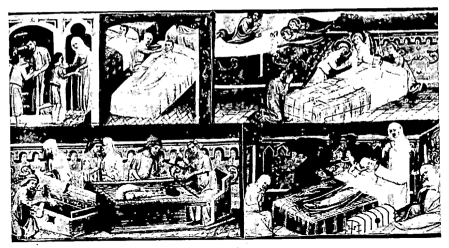

Early fourteenth century French hospital scenes.

intellectual decline and made few contributions to medicine. While herbal remedies were used by monks for everyday disorders, it was felt that life on earth was merely a brief interim before the heavenly reward. Suffering was seen as a means to salvation, practical branches of medicine like surgery were regarded as lowly, and dissection was banned.

In the twelfth century secular medicine began to emerge again. It stemmed from the School of Salerno where scholars began to translate some of the original medical texts of Galen and Hippocrates. The Church, however, imposed strict controls on how medicine should develop.

Christianity did leave one permanent legacy to medicine, however — the hospital system. Care of the poor, and in particular the sick and the homeless, was an integral part of Christian teaching. Starting with guest houses set aside for pilgrims, many hospitals were created including in London St Bartholomews, which was founded in the twelfth century, and St Thomas's, founded less than a century later. A number of hospitals had provision for women in childbed.

The Renaissance

By the middle of the fifteenth century there were signs that medicine was emerging from the torpor into which it had slumped. Constraints imposed by the Christian Church ceased to be effective, and there was a new freedom of intellect.

Fundamental to the 'rebirth' or Renaissance was an interest in the Greeks and Romans, their buildings, thoughts and their concern for and love of the human body. Painters were in the vanguard of this movement,

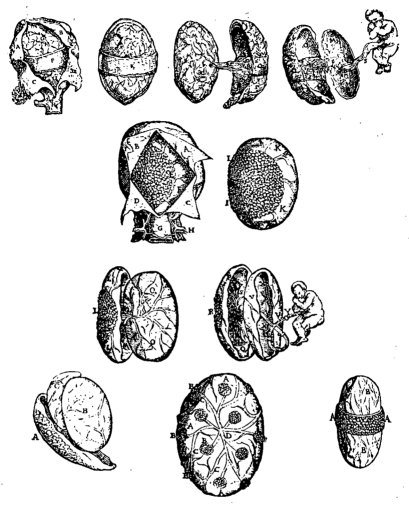

Diagram of the uterus by Vesalius. (Humani Corporis fabrica, 1542)

and their desire to represent the human body faithfully led men like Leonardo da Vinci to take an interest in dissection. In 1543 Vesalius published his revolutionary *The Fabric of the Human Body*, insisting that the truth could be reached only by dissection and study of human bodies. His work revealed errors in Galen's teaching, and after its appearance reliance on Galen as the ultimate authority began to wane.

The new scientific study of anatomy was also directed towards the process of childbirth, which had been largely ignored during the mediaeval period. For the first time the accurate form of the gravid (pregnant) uterus was illustrated by Leonardo. Stimulated by the work of Vesalius, other men made real steps towards an understanding of

99

women's diseases and the mechanics of labour. Precise descriptions of the
female anatomy were drawn up based on accurate observation rather
than on theories handed down from classical times.

Surgical techniques in childbirth had made no advance in the mediaeval
period and were still limited to the destructive operations which had been
carried out in extremis throughout recorded history. In early western society
Caesarean section was primarily important because it allowed the child to
be buried separately. In 1500 there was a notable — if isolated — event in
this area. Joseph Nufer, a sow gelder, called in midwives and doctors
when his wife ran into trouble during labour. When none of the
attendants proved able to help, Nufer himself peformed a Caesarean and
delivered a living baby. His wife recovered too, and lived to be seventy-
seven and have six more children naturally.

Despite Nufer's success, it was to be many centuries before Caesarean
section was considered as an operation that could be performed on a
dying mother when the child showed signs of life, or on a living mother
in an effort to save both mother and child. During the sixteenth century,
however, a major advance in obstetrics was made with the reintroduction
of podalic version by the French barber-surgeon, Ambroise Paré, who
had trained at the Hotel Dieu. Version had been known since ancient
times and used by some midwives, but Paré was the first to give a precise
description of how it could be performed.

The late fifteenth century suffered the outbreak of a new and dreadful
disease, different from the plagues and epidemics which had punctuated
European history. It was characterised by skin eruptions and ulcerations
which caused widespread destruction of tissue and resulted in many
deaths. It was believed to have been brought to Naples by the sailors of
Christopher Columbus, and at various times was dubbed the 'Spanish',
'French' and the 'Neopolitan' disease. During the sixteenth century its
origin was found to be venereal, and it was named 'Syphilis' by Girolamo
Fracastoro. His book *De Contagione*, published in 1546, was an attempt
to bring some order to the huge body of material that had been amassed
on the disease, and it represented a new attitude to medicine. It was the
first complete observation of the spread of infections, and a revision of
the Hippocratic method of observing symptoms.

The seventeenth century

In the seventeenth century it was clearly France which was leading the
field in obstetrics. The Hotel Dieu saw the delivery of over one hundred
babies a month and trainees saw more deliveries than a medical student
could hope to see today. This, and the increasing fame of surgeons
following in the steps of Ambroise Paré, ensured that every enterprising
doctor wanting to study midwifery went to Paris.

The Hotel Dieu's greatest pupil was François Mauriceau whose book, *Traité des maladies des femmes grosses et celles qui sont accouchées*, published in 1668, was founded on practical experience and offered realistic advice; this book and a companion volume offered the first rational base for the art of midwifery. Mauriceau, Jacques Guillemeau (Paré's favourite pupil) and other men who had been trained at the Hotel Dieu were essentially responsible for bringing midwifery within the province of the male accoucheur.

In Britain at this time the man midwife was called in primarily to perform surgery, but the invention of the forceps by the Chamberlen brothers was to reinforce the increasing importance of the male attendant. The seventeenth century also saw the first original book on midwifery published in Britain. William Harvey's *De Generatione Animalium* came out in 1651 and has earned the author the title of 'the Father of British Midwifery'.[2] The book was important because it was based on his own observations rather than relying on the evidence of past authorities. Among his many observations, Harvey noted the large open area, which he likened to an open wound, which was left in the womb after the delivery of the placenta, and he mentioned cases of high fever with an offensive lochial discharge which sometimes followed an apparently normal delivery — probably cases of puerperal fever. In normal birth Harvey urged patience, watchfulness, gentleness and as little interference in nature as possible.

Percival Willughby, the man midwife, was a friend of Harvey's. He was another believer in the 'invisible midwife, Dame Nature':

> The midwife's duty in a natural birth is no more but to attend and wait on Nature, and to receive the child, and (if need require) to help to fetch the afterbirth, and her best care will be Nature's servant. Let them always remember that gentle proceedings (with moderate warm-keeping, and having their endeavours dulcified with sweet words) will best erase and relieve and soonest deliver their labouring women.[3]

Willughby saw many instances of malpractice on the part of midwives — male and female. He described many of his fellow practitioners as inexperienced surgeons or ill-prepared apothecaries who, 'leaving the beating of their mortars, turn Doctors as also taking it upon themselves to be men midwives'[4] and berated those who used 'pothooks, pack-needles, silver spoons, thatcher's knives'.[5] To avoid such horrors he undertook to instruct his daughters in midwifery himself.

Developments in midwifery apart, the seventeenth century was the age of scientific revolution and saw the introduction of many new sciences — higher mathematics, astronomy, physics and chemistry. All of these affected medicine as throughout Europe researchers took new directions to fill the gaps left by the demolition of Galenic teaching. The major medical progress came through the development of physiology, the study of how the living body works. In 1628, for example, William Harvey, studying the flow of blood, discovered valves in the veins which allow the blood to pass only in one direction. From this he drew the conclusion that the blood which was being continuously pumped into the arteries must be the same blood which was returning through the veins. In other words, the blood circulated. The Royal Society in London, founded by scholars and scientists to promote progress, championed Harvey's theory of circulation, and began also to use microscopes extensively for physiological research. Three members of the Royal Society, Christopher Wren, Robert Boyle and Richard Lower were also responsible for the first successful blood transfusion — although after a number of disasters, investigations into the technique were abandoned and not revived until the nineteenth century.

The need to devise new treatments for disease had been made particularly acute in the seventeenth century because of the ravages caused by the plague, which proved resistant to all treatments attempted by physicians. The only way to avoid it seemed to be to escape to the fresh air of the country. Although the plague of 1665 did not return after the Great Fire of London in 1666 which cleansed the city, the almost total ignorance of personal and public hygiene remained a constant hazard to health.

The eighteenth century — the new midwifery

In 1726 a bizarre case attracted public attention. A woman called Maria Tofts, while sitting in a field, had been frightened by a rabbit. Soon after, she claimed to have given birth to a rabbit, and then to many more. Soon people were flocking to see the event. A man midwife, John Howard, was called in to attend the births, and the court sent a representative who confirmed the strange occurrence. Only months later was Maria Tofts exposed as a fraud by Sir Richard Manningham, a leading man midwife.

The case is revealing of the eighteenth century, not because the fraud was discovered, but because it was by no means dismissed as an impossibility even in London society. Above all the eighteenth century was the age of quackery, and childbirth was already so shrouded in strange beliefs that anything was possible.

In France, the development of hospital schools gave doctors the clinical training they had lacked before. By the eighteenth century a number of techniques were being developed to measure the birth passage so that there was prior warning of any difficulties that might arise. The clinical observation of birth finally removed it from the realm of magic and superstition and gave obstetrics a scientific basis; but in fact there

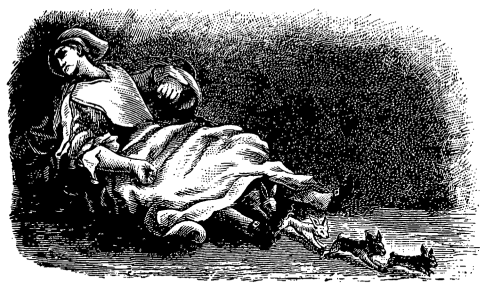

Maria Tofts, giving birth to rabbits. (Engraving by William Hogarth)

was little that could be done to assist a woman with complications when version was not enough. Attempts were made to enlarge the birth canal with deep cuts, or to open the abdomen, but they were usually calamitous. Although instrumental delivery, in the hands of the untrained practitioner could be, and often was, disastrous, the fusion of the French study of pelvimetry and British advances in surgery resulted in a 'New Midwifery' that began to make obstetrics effective and ensured the survival of many women and babies who would otherwise have died.

In 1739 a Scot, William Smellie, travelled south from Lanark. He had trained in Glasgow and Paris, then settled in London, where he became the leading man midwife. Described by an opponent as a 'rawboned large-handed man no more fit for the business than a ploughman is fit for a dancing master',[6] he was nevertheless the acknowledged master of British midwifery. During his years in London his classes were attended by 900 students and he attended 1150 labours.

When demonstrating to his pupils, Smellie used a 'machine' and a dummy on which to demonstrate the different forms of presentation and how to deal with them. At this time a man midwife had to deliver babies under a sheet or with a cloth between him and the mother. Smellie used forceps when he considered it necessary, but he was fond of holding up a pair of rusty old forceps to show his students how infrequently they had been used. Out of 1000 deliveries, he claimed to have required instruments only ten times. He believed that it required more skill to avoid than to perform obstetric operations, a belief much quoted by James Young Simpson, one of the greatest obstetricians of the nineteenth century. In a difficult delivery, where instrumental intervention was required, he preferred the forceps to the lever or fillet, because he thought they did less damage to the child. At first he used wooden forceps to mask the noise they made, well aware of the prejudice and fear which surrounded them. Later he replaced them with metallic ones covered with leather so that they did not clink. Even so, his forceps were only eleven inches long and were used when the baby's head was well down in the pelvis.

Smellie's *Treatise on Midwifery* was published in 1752 with the help of the novelist Tobias Smollett who had been one of his students. It gives a clear account of the mechanism of labour, corrects many errors and lays down sensible rules for obstetrical practice. Smellie was the first person to publish an illustration of a pelvis deformed by rickets, and he developed his own technique for pelvic measurement which was simple, practical and dependable. He also stressed the importance of the relationship between pelvic contraction and the size of the baby. He believed there were very few cases when contraction was so bad that the baby could not be brought out alive.

Smellie's French counterpart was André Levret. He was such a popular teacher that students travelled from all over Europe to study under him. Much of Levret's work was done on the pelvis, but he also made a number of alterations to forceps already in use, and invented some with a pelvic curve. Both Smellie and Levret wanted to see the forceps improved. Much of the groundwork for improvement had already been done by Edmund Chapman, William Giffard and Benjamin Pugh, who had been using and modifying forceps for a number of years before the design of the Chamberlen forceps was made public.

In 1754 Pugh published his *Treatise on Midwifery*. He disapproved of women lying on their backs for delivery, especially when there were complications. Instead he advised standing, kneeling or, best of all, sitting on a pillow on the lap of a strong woman in an armchair. Using either podalic version or forceps, he delivered all his patients successfully 'without opening one child's head for these fourteen years past'.[7]

Another Scot, William Hunter, was to command a leading position in obstetrics. Hunter arrived in London in 1740, and lived with Smellie for nearly a year. He studied and later taught anatomy. In 1749 he was appointed surgeon midwife to the British Lying-in Hospital and he held a similar position at the Middlesex Hospital. He was anxious to establish hospitals for lying-in women and determined to promote the acceptance of the man midwife despite the opposition of doctors and midwives. Hunter was very popular at court, and this was an advantage in his quest to make obstetrics respectable. He was first called in to attend the confinement of George III's queen, Charlotte, although the actual delivery was made by the midwife, Mrs Draper.

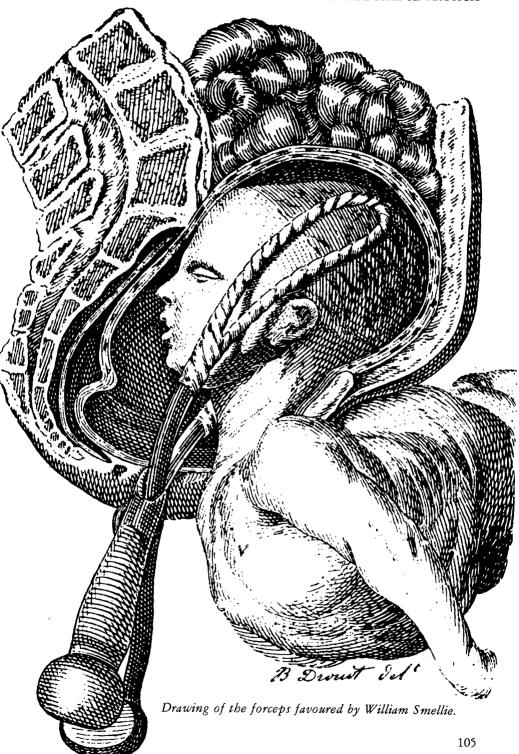

Drawing of the forceps favoured by William Smellie.

Hunter was liked for his kindness and his charm, and the confidence he inspired, and so successful was he that he bought a house in Great Windmill Street where he built a large museum, lecture theatre and dissecting rooms. All his important contributions to obstetrics were anatomical, and although he was unable to make the Royal College of Physicians accept men midwives, his influence at court and his eminence in anatomy and obstetrics generally helped to raise it from a despised craft to a special discipline.

In Ireland, the first important teacher of midwifery was Fielding Ould. In 1748 he had published his *Treatise of Midwifery* which was important primarily for his study of the mechanism of labour. He was ahead of his time in prescribing opiates for women undergoing a difficult labour. He was also the first to advise an episiotomy when the perineum looked as if it would tear. Caesarean section he regarded as a 'detestable, barbarous, illegal piece of inhumanity'.[8]

In France around this time the field was led by 'Le Grand Baudeloque', Jean Louis Baudeloque. Napoleon summoned him for the first confinement of the Empress Marie Louise, and he was Professor of the Paris Maternité from 1797 to 1810. Baudeloque showed how contraction of the pelvis could be revealed through external measurements. Up until this time, the usual means of measurement had been a compass, the legs of which were inserted into the pelvic area. His new methods were an advance not only because they were less painful, but because they allowed women to maintain the new-found standards of modesty. Baudeloque was one of the few obstetricians of the eighteenth century to advocate Caesarean section in cases where the pelvis was badly contracted. He was branded an assassin for his belief, but he reported on thirty-one successful cases collected from numerous sources from 1750 onwards.

Various attempts at Caesarean section were made in Britain in the eighteenth century, with little success. One exception was noted by Smellie: an illiterate Irish woman, Mary Donally, 'emminent among the common people for extracting dead births'[9] saved both mother and baby in 1738. Donally had used a sharp razor to make an incision to the side of the midline of the belly. She then:

> held the lips of the wound together with her hand, till one went a
> mile and returned with silk and cotton needles which tailors used.
> With these she joined the lips in the manner of the stitch employed
> ordinarily for the hare lip, and dressed the wound with whites of
> eggs.[10]

In 1740 another operation for dealing with severe pelvic contraction, symphisiotomy, had been proposed to the Royal Academy in France by Jean Renée Sigault. In 1777 he performed the operation successfully, but the patient was rendered incontinent. The complications inherent in the

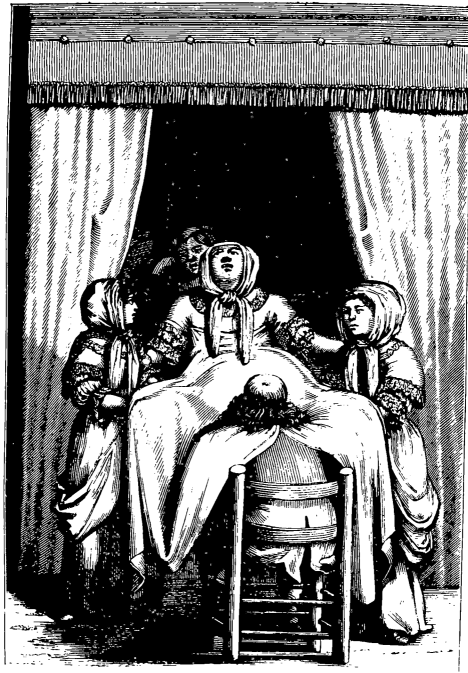

*When a woman was delivered by a man she often had to be delivered under a
sheet because of the constraints of modesty. (Engraving by Abraham Bosse)*

operation meant that it never became popular and was only revived at the end of the nineteenth century.

That Caesarean section was not completely abandoned was due in large part to the efforts of Manchester surgeons Charles White and John Hull, who did a great deal to establish the operation as necessary and justifiable in cases of gross deformity of the pelvis. Craniotomy, though, continued to be adhered to by most British surgeons until the end of the nineteenth century.

None of the advances of obstetrics could be of real value, however, until the problem of puerperal fever was solved.

In 1772 the worst epidemic of fever broke out and decimated women in hospitals all over Europe. That year also saw the publication of a book by Charles White of Manchester, in which he described the customary practices following birth:

> As soon as she is delivered, if she be a person in affluent circumstances, she is covered up close in bed with additional clothes, the curtains are drawn round the bed and pinned together, every crevice in the windows and doors is stuffed close, not excepting even the keyhole . . . and the good woman is not suffered to put her arm or even her nose, out of bed for fear of catching cold. She is constantly supplied out of the spout of a teapot with large quantities of warm liquors, to keep up perspiration and sweat, and her whole diet consists of them. She is confined to the horizontal position for many days together, whereby both the stools and the lochia are prevented from having a free exit. . . . The lochia, stagnating in the womb and the folds of the vagina, soon grow putrid. . . .[11]

White denounced such practices, and advocated revolutionary techniques such as adequate ventilation and scrupulous cleanliness on the part of all attendants as well as of towels, bed linen and instruments. He suggested that women should be allowed to take cold or tepid baths during pregnancy and after birth, that the child should be allowed to make its own way out during birth, and that the cord should not be severed immediately. Most revolutionary of all, he believed that after birth a woman should be placed in as upright a position as possible so that the uterus could drain. Further, she should be allowed to get up as soon as she was able, usually on the second day. Most importantly, White displayed a clear understanding of the relationship between the infection following surgery in a crowded hospital and puerperal fever, but despite the clarity of his suggestions, opinion about the actual cause of the fever continued to be divided in medical circles.

In Vienna, Dr Lucas Johann Boer, professor of midwifery and director of the lying-in hospital, was greatly impressed by White's work. He refused to teach midwifery on the female cadaver, using a leather model instead. Unfortunately, after his retirement his methods were soon neglected.

In Scotland, meanwhile, study of the nature of puerperal fever had been furthered by Alexander Gordon in Aberdeen. In 1775 he published his *Treatise on the Epidemic Puerperal Fever of Aberdeen*, which clearly indicated the infectious nature of the fever. Gordon demonstrated that the fever was not a 'miasma' in the air as was commonly believed, because the fever was not indiscriminate but was suffered only by a woman visited or delivered by a practitioner or nurse who had previously attended a patient with the fever. He produced a table showing how different attendants had infected different patients. Puerperal fever was infectious like smallpox or measles. Because of this he did not feel that ventilation or cleanliness would destroy the infection, and advocated more stringent precautions like fumigation of wards, clothing and bedding. Neither White's nor Gordon's preventive measures was generally adopted. As a result epidemics continued to break out nearly every year.

While no decisive advances were made in medicine, the problems of disease and infection had, by the eighteenth century, if anything worsened. Sanitation was particularly bad in the towns where

> city ditches, now often filled with stagnant water, were commonly used as latrines; butchers killed animals in their shops and threw the offal of the carcases into the streets; dead animals were left to decay and fester where they lay; latrine pits were dug close to wells, thus contaminating the water supply. Decomposing bodies of the rich in burial vaults beneath the church often stank out parson and congregation; urban cemeteries became overcrowded as the population grew, and the decaying bodies, constantly disturbed to make way for others, began to pollute the air of the neighbourhood.[12]

The consequences for health were disastrous. There were outbursts of dysentery, intestinal worms were common, malarial fevers were rife in poorly drained marsh areas, and tuberculosis was a common cause of death. Once the plague had subsided, however, the most feared disease was smallpox. It affected all of society, rich and poor, and when it did not kill it left many survivors blind, pockmarked and disfigured for life.

Inoculation against smallpox had been known in the Far East for centuries. It was accomplished by opening a vein and inserting a needle containing some of the pox. The technique was introduced into Britain in the eighteeenth century by Lady Mary Wortley Montague, the wife of the British Ambassador in Constantinople, where inoculation was commonplace. The method had marked success, but was not without risk. In 1796 Edward Jenner, an English country doctor, discovered how the risk could be reduced without a significant loss of protection. He began to inoculate patients with cowpox, a disease of the udders of cows, which gave recipients the necessary protection without the dangers. His discovery was a medical breakthrough: but Jenner could not explain how it worked.

Probably the greatest development made in the eighteenth century was the reawakening of interest in public health. Some towns began to attempt to deal with the problems of sanitation, and the importance of good ventilation began to gain credence through the work of men like Black, Priestley and Lavoisier. In the navy, John Lind stressed the need for a balanced diet for sailors, and an army physician, Sir John Pringle, noted that the epidemic fevers which ravaged troops rarely broke out in camps which were well spaced and open.

With the growing urbanisation of the population from the mid-eighteenth century there was an increased demand for food, the country became better cultivated and drained, and there were many improvements in agricultural techniques. But industrialisation had a far-reaching effect on city life. Overcrowding, squalor and poverty in the towns and cities held up the effective implementation of public health measures until the twentieth century.

In the meantime, however, medicine began to be effective for the first time.

The nineteenth century — Medicine becomes effective

During the eighteenth century there had, then, been a constant probing of ideas and problems. A clearer understanding of the mechanics of labour had been reached and attention had been focused on puerperal fever. At the beginning of the nineteenth century, however, amputation of the breast was practically the only operation carried out regularly to treat the particular ills of women.

In 1809 an American called Ephraim McDowell, who had trained in Edinburgh, performed an ovariotomy on a woman called Jane Crawford in Kentucky. The operation was carried out without anaesthetic and it took twenty-five minutes — but it was successful. Other doctors followed McDowell's example, and by the middle of the century

the first major gynaecological operation had been undertaken by a dozen men in different parts of the world and was beginning to be accepted, though still with some misgivings, as a surgical procedure which despite its high mortality was occasionally necessary.[13]

Pioneering work similar to McDowell's was performed by two more Americans. In 1827 John Lambert Richmond, forced by circumstances to rely on his own initiative, performed the second Caesarean section of the nineteenth century. Using a pocket knife he performed this operation on a black woman lying on a kitchen table. His technique, however, differed very little from that described by Scipione Mercurio in 1596 and did not offer any real solution to the problems inherent in performing a Caesarean. The other American was Marion Sims, who was responsible

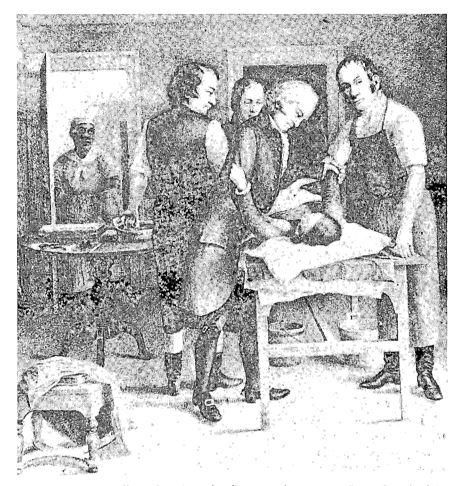

Ephraim McDowell performing the first ovariotomy on Jane Crawford in Danville, Kentucky, December 1809. The patient, strapped to the kitchen table, recited the psalms to keep up her spirits.

for a real breakthrough in gynaecological surgery: the repair of the vesico-vaginal fistula, an unpleasant and quite common problem. The vesico-vaginal fistula is a tear between the bladder and the vagina, and is usually caused either by a very prolonged and difficult labour or by bad midwifery. As a result, urine leaks through into the vagina, and if the wound does not heal itself, the unfortunate sufferer would be doomed to a life of discomfort and isolation. Sims' reputation was made on the basis of his cure, and he moved to New York where he continued his work and opened a hospital — the first of its kind — specifically for the treatment of the diseases peculiar to women.

By the end of the century, thanks to a combination of skill on the part of surgeons and to the introduction of anaesthesia, it had become possible to remove ovarian cysts and fibroids, to deal with ectopic pregnancies, perform hysterectomies and repair fistulae. The groundwork for the establishment of gynaecology as a speciality had been laid.

Obstetrics – problems and progress

Obstetrics in the nineteenth century lagged behind gynaecology. There were many advances in the field, but they did not necessarily benefit the nineteenth-century woman; and in some instances discoveries in inept hands could be a real danger.

Ergot, for example, began to be used widely for the stimulation of labour. Ergot had been used for this purpose by midwives for centuries, but the first scientific report on ergot was not until 1774. After the publication of a paper in New York in 1822 by John Stearns, it began to be widely used by the medical profession, and by the end of the century it was commonly used to stop post-partum haemorrhage and to speed up labour.

Stearns had warned that ergot should only be used in certain groups of cases, but it quickly began to be used as a matter of routine, and was much abused. No antidote was known, and used without care it could cause the uterus to rupture, mould around the baby and kill it, or prevent expulsion of the placenta.

The greatest barrier to improving on the high maternal mortality statistics in childbirth remained puerperal fever. Despite the work of White and Gordon, few doctors were willing to admit that they themselves could be carriers of contagion. By the mid-century, however, a more thorough understanding of its cause, together with preventive measures for its control, had been suggested by an American, Oliver Wendell Holmes, and a Hungarian, Ignaz Semmelweis.

Holmes became interested in the subject after hearing of a physician who had performed a post-mortem on a woman who had died of the fever. Soon afterwards, the doctor himself had died, but before his death he had attended other women in childbirth, all of whom had contracted puerperal fever. Holmes began to amass facts about the fever, and his findings were published in April 1843.[14] He reiterated the belief that the fever was often transmitted by doctors and other attendants. He insisted that anyone who had conducted a post-mortem, attended a case of the fever or a case of erysipelas could be an agent responsible for infecting the next patient he saw. To stop this contagion Holmes recommended that all doctors involved in midwifery should abstain from actively taking part in post-mortems or dissections. Even if a doctor was only an attendant at a case, he should wash thoroughly, change his clothes and allow some

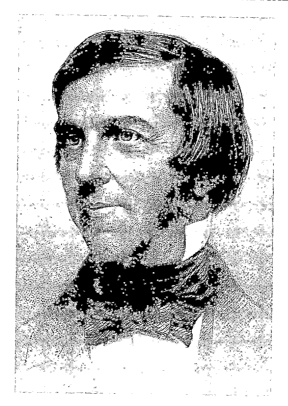

Oliver Wendell Holmes, the American physician who produced evidence of the infectious nature of puerperal fever and advocated measures to prevent its spread.

time to elapse before he attended a childbed. The same caution should be employed after attending a case of erysipelas. If it became clear that fever was present in a practice, the doctor concerned should stop practising for at least a month and, if necessary, longer. Holmes maintained:

> . . . the time has come when the existence of a private pestilence in the sphere of a single physician should be looked upon, not as a misfortune, but a crime.[15]

Holmes was bitterly criticised, in particular for his suggestion that physicians could be carriers of disease. His reply was compelling:

> I take no offence and attempt no retort. No man can quarrel with me over the counterpane that covers a mother with the new-born infant at her breast.[16]

Among the evidence that Holmes presented to support his theory were the findings of Ignaz Semmelweis; and Semmelweis it was who discovered how the infection was transmitted.

Semmelweis worked in the Vienna Lying-in Hospital where in 1839 Lucas Boer had been succeeded by Johann Klein. Klein abandoned Boer's teaching methods and taught in dissecting rooms and he and his students would go straight from there to attend a woman in labour. In his first year as a professor, the incidence of puerperal fever soared. A colleague in the hospital, Kolletschka, was accidentally cut while performing a post-mortem. Septicaemia set in and he died soon after; but Semmelweis noted that the course and development of the infection was remarkably similar to that of puerperal fever. He drew parallels: his colleague's cut, the extensive internal wound suffered by a woman where the placenta has separated. She, examined by a student, was as likely to pick up 'cadaveric material' from the dissecting rooms as Kolletschka had been.

In May 1847 Semmelweis introduced a rigid regime of cleanliness, and all students had to scrub their hands in a solution of chloride of lime before delivering, examining or touching a patient. By the end of 1847 the death rate in his wards had fallen dramatically, and he was now convinced that:

> Puerperal fever is caused by conveyance to the pregnant woman of putrid articles derived from living organisms, through the agency of the examining fingers.[17]

He also admitted cases of self-infection could occur when, for example, part of the placenta remained or decomposed in the body. Sadly, most men of science ignored his work and did not implement his recommended procedures to eliminate the chances of infection. Conditions in many hospitals remained appalling. When Leon Le Fort visited the Paris Maternité in 1864 he wrote:

> The principal ward contained a large number of beds in alcoves like English horse-stalls along each side. Ventilation was almost impossible. Floors and partitions were washed perhaps once a month . . . the ceilings had not been white-washed for many a long year. Lying-in women who became ill were transferred to an isolation room regardless of the nature of the illness — puerperal fever cases and patients affected with diarrhoea, bronchitis, measles, or any other eruptive fever. Midwife pupils attend normal lying-in patients and fever cases alike, and perform all the necessary manipulations for every class of case.[18]

As Le Fort went on to say

> It is not astonishing that the Maternité of Paris has furnished a mortality without example in any European country. From 1860 to 1864 the patients numbered 9,886, of whom 1,226 died, equal to a mortality of 12.4 per cent.[19]

Despite the opposition to it, Semmelweis's work still saved thousands of

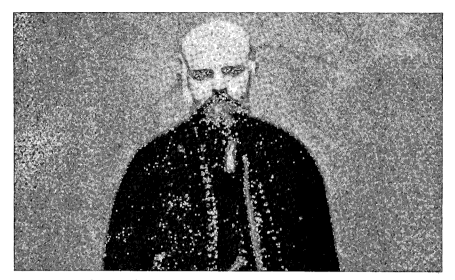

Ignaz Semmelweiss, the Hungarian doctor whose work in Vienna established the cause of puerperal fever.

lives. Ironically, he died from the very infection he had devoted most of his life to preventing.

A number of further advances were made during the second half of the nineteenth century. There was a lessening of resistance to instruments like the speculum, the uterine sound and other new and improved curettes and dilators. Gradually they became increasingly important to the obstetrician. Although there were still many misconceptions about the female reproductive system, advances had been made in this area too; but the mechanisms that triggered the onset of menstruation and the monthly cycle were not understood until the twentieth century. The effects of tuberculosis on a pregnant woman began to be understood, and the theory that pregnancy improved the health of a tubercular woman was dispelled.

Eclampsia remained a very real threat, but in 1843 Lever of Guy's Hospital in London discovered albumin in the urine of his patients, and Simpson made similar observations. In 1896 a paper on the treatment of eclampsia was read in the Rotunda in Dublin. It recommended the use of morphia, venesection, purgation and oxygen if necessary. No food or drugs were to be given by mouth in an attack, and the patient was to be placed on her side so that any secretion would flow out of her mouth instead of into the lungs. Induction of labour was condemned, and delivery could be speeded up only if the cervix showed signs of dilation.

A better technique for delivery of the placenta was also introduced. In 1853 Carl Siegmund Franz Credé developed a method of expressing the placenta by massaging the uterus for fifteen to thirty minutes after the delivery of the baby. He began very gently and gradually increased the amount of compression until the placenta was expelled naturally.

Furious debate still raged over the use of Caesarean section for much of the century, and in the meantime the most common obstetric operations remained craniotomy and version. Improvements in instruments were made, and variations and modification to the forceps were also under constant review.

Version reached new heights in 1860 when Braxton Hicks reintroduced bipolar version, a technique similar to that introduced by Mercurio centuries earlier. Hicks combined external and internal manipulations to alter the position of the baby, inserting two fingers rather than the whole hand while the other hand manipulated externally. It was very effective even when internal version had failed. Hicks was also responsible for identifying the contractions which occur at intervals throughout pregnancy and which have been named after him.

Medicine and understanding

Although the nineteenth century was important for the establishment and consolidation of gynaecology and obstetrics as specialities, these are inextricably linked with — and would have been impossible without — advances made in medicine and society as a whole.

At the beginning of the century ideas about disease and its treatment were not vastly different from those of Ancient Greece. Physicians still did not really know what caused disease and had no new treatments for it, despite the discoveries in anatomy and physiology. Surgeons, too, were still hampered by the age-old problems of pain, bleeding and infection. As in other centuries, progress must be attributed to the discoveries made by individual men and women who realised the importance of details which others had missed. However, the development of the sciences which were both a cause and a result of the Industrial Revolution gave these people advantages which had not been available before.

Chemistry and physics were two of these sciences. Although their impetus was the development of the new textile and engineering industries, they were soon to prove invaluable to medical researchers also. Chemists were now able to produce and analyse a whole range of different chemicals and to study their effects on the human body. From here it was only a step to the development of biochemistry and the study and analysis of the human body's own chemical substances.

Many other advances were also to prove a boon to medicine. Optical instrument makers laid the groundwork for the development of more powerful microscopes to study diseases and their effects on humans, paving the way for men like Konrad von Röntgen who discovered the X-

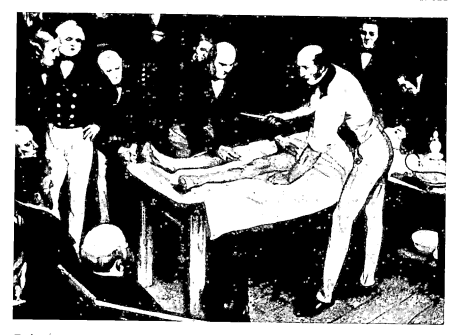

Robert Liston, the British surgeon, performing the first operation using anaesthesia in Britain, 21 December 1846. In the background, extreme left, is the young Joseph Lister, who later pioneered antisepsis.

ray. Engineers and technicians produced more precise and delicate instruments which could be used to equal advantage by surgeons. Revolution in communications in the form of railways and the telegraph opened up the availability of information. Even the ill effects of industrialisation played a part. The serious epidemics of disease which killed thousands of people living in overcrowded and squalid urban conditions eventually forced governments to realise that improvements in sanitation and public health generally must be instigated.

Surgery

At the beginning of the nineteenth century the surgeon's skills were based on his knowledge of the anatomy, his skill with the knife, and speed. James Young Simpson described how Robert Liston, the surgeon, 'operated with such speed that the sound of sawing seemed to succeed immediately the first flash of the knife'.[20] Yet the sleight of hand which made limb surgery possible was often not enough. Patients had to be dragged screaming from the wards and held down by grim force until the leather belts had been buckled tightly over their writhing bodies. In

117

addition to the pain and shock involved, the flagrant disregard for the most basic hygiene was a major hurdle, infection was rampant, and wounds often festered and reopened, causing secondary haemorrhage.

Anaesthesia

By the beginning of the nineteenth century experiments were under way with some of the new chemicals and gases to find a substance more powerful than opium to dull the pain suffered by patients. Sir Humphrey Davy and Michael Faraday experimented with nitrous oxide or laughing gas, but nothing came of their findings. However, in America in the 1840s four men, Crawford Long, Horace Wells, William Morton and Charles Jackson, were also experimenting with various substances. In 1845 Horace Wells gave a public demonstration of what was meant to be painless tooth extraction using nitrous oxide. The attempt was a failure, but in 1846 at the Massachusetts General Hospital, William Morton successfully removed a tumour from a patient using ether. News of this success quickly spread to Britain, and in the same year Robert Liston successfully amputated a leg using ether. As he remarked, 'this Yankee dodge, gentlemen, beats mesmerism hollow'.[21] Ether soon proved to have its disadvantages because it irritated the lungs and became unstable when exposed to air. However, there was another substance: chloroform.
On 4 November 1847, in Edinburgh, James Young Simpson and some friends decided to experiment on themselves with choloroform. On awakening from the unconsciousness which it produced, it is reported that Simpson's first thought was, 'this is far stronger and better than ether'.[22] Before two weeks had passed he had administered chloroform to fifty patients with good results.
Simpson is rightly famous for his discovery and use of chloroform. He was also one of the outstanding figures in obstetrics of the nineteenth century. But the introduction of anaesthesia was, in a way, a two-edged sword. In childbirth it gave relief to many women, but it also led to other, more barbaric obstetric operations gaining popularity in some countries; many operations which before the introduction of anaesthesia had been impossible now became an option. There was an outbreak of *Accouchement Forcé* — the polite name given to violent delivery whatever the risk. In cases where the cervix was slow to dilate, of eclampsia, accidental haemorrhage or even placenta praevia, the cervix was often forcibly dilated. Sometimes dilation was discarded altogether and incisions were made in the cervical canal to reach the uterus and force the baby's head through. Such operations caused severe damage to the uterus and maternal mortality from haemorrhage; shock and sepsis were high, and infant mortality even higher. Symphysiotomy and pubiotomy

enjoyed a new vogue. Most of these techniques, however, fell into disuse at the end of the century when Caesarean section finally became viable.

Techniques of Caesarean section had remained largely unchanged until well into the 1870s. Until that time it was still widely believed that it was not necessary to suture the uterine wall. In 1872 a British doctor, Fleetwood Churchill, wrote:

> No sutures are required in the uterus, as it contracts the wound will
> be reduced to about 1-2 inches and the lips will come into apposition,
> if it be healthy.[23]

In 1876 Eduardo Porro managed to overcome many of the problems inherent in the operation by performing a hysterectomy following a section. This considerably reduced the risk of haemorrhage and sepsis, but it was a very extreme solution. Meanwhile, gynaecological surgeons like Lawson Tait in England were beginning to report successes with suturing the wall of the uterus. The real breakthrough came when this technique was applied following a Caesarean by F A Kehrer and Max Sanger in 1881 and 1882 respectively. Sanger, using aseptic methods and

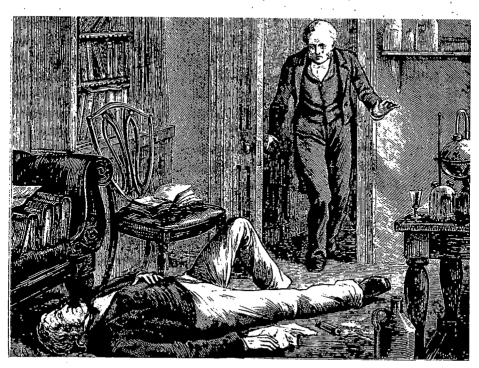

James Young Simpson experimenting on himself with chloroform. Sir Walter Scott later suggested that an appropriate coat of arms for Simpson would be 'a wee naked bairn' with the motto, 'Does your mother know you're out?'

119

Even so, a more effective way of stopping shock following haemorrhage was urgently needed, and the most obvious solution was to replace the blood lost by the patient. Experiments in transfusion had been attempted since the seventeenth century using direct transfusion from one animal to another and from an animal to a human, but there were problems of clotting, and many patients died for no apparent reason. By 1900 Karl Landsteiner of Vienna had been able to show that there were different blood groups which could not be safely transfused into one another, but it was only in the twentieth century that transfusion became viable.

Infection

Real medical advance became possible when the connection between disease, dirt and the spread of infection began to be understood. As early as 1683 Anthony van Leuwenhoek in Amsterdam had seen bacteria under a single lens microscope, but in the early nineteenth century it was still widely believed that bacteria were the result of disease, not its cause. An initial breakthrough came when in the mid-nineteenth century scientists began to suggest that decay might be caused by airborne microbes. Eventually in 1864 Louis Pasteur in France was able to show convincingly how these microbes caused decay.

In the 1870s work in the same field was being carried out by a German, Robert Koch. After studying anthrax germs in animals, Koch went on to study infection of the human body. In 1878 he identified germs causing blood poisoning and septicaemia in wounds, and it was during these researches that he devised one of the most important experimental techniques for studying disease. Because he often had difficulty in seeing the germs in the blood affected by septicaemia — even when he knew they were there — he began staining them with a dye called methyl violet. The staining technique was to become critically important later in the search for antibacterial agents.

In the wake of the pioneering work of men like Koch and Pasteur, the organisms of at least twenty-one diseases were discovered, including two which had a real impact on obstetric practices. Gonorrhoea had long been a very real hazard to a new-born baby. If the mother had the disease, the baby's eyes were affected as the child passed down the birth canal. In 1884, following the discovery of the coccus responsible for the disease Credé came up with a means of preventing such cases of blindness, recommending bathing the eyes of the newborn with clean water and applying a single drop of a two per cent solution of silver nitrate to the middle of the cornea. His simple remedy saved the sight of thousands of children.

The haemolytic streptococcus, the bacteria which causes puerperal fever, was also identified, and the work of Semmelweis and Holmes vindicated. Pasteur and others had identified germs in the lochia of infected mothers in the 1860s, but in 1879 Pasteur managed to culture the bacteria and systematically linked the microbe to the infection. Because of the virulence of the microbe, the only real weapon was total hygiene. The pioneer in this field was Joseph Lister. Reading of Pasteur's work, Lister realised the effect that micro-organisms carried in the air must have on wounds, and he set up a means of destroying the microbes by thorough cleansing with carbolic acid. Instruments were kept in carbolic acid, and for the operation itself he invented a pump which sprayed the air with carbolic. The number of patients dying from the infection dropped dramatically. However, because the micro-organisms could not be seen with the naked eye, many doctors and medical attendants failed to carry out his aseptic techniques, which they regarded as too much trouble.

It was only in the 1890s that the importance of Lister's work was widely accepted. Scientists, now able to culture bacteria, began to test carbolic acid to see just how effective it was at killing germs, and concluded that where dirt or germs existed, antiseptics were often ineffectual because the bacteria could protect themselves in the dirt. The important thing was to exclude microbes from the area being operated on rather than trying to kill them once they were present. Aseptic practices were introduced — dressings were exposed to steam, instruments boiled, and surgical processes made as sterile as possible. In 1890 W S Halstead, an American surgeon, introduced rubber gloves to give even further protection.

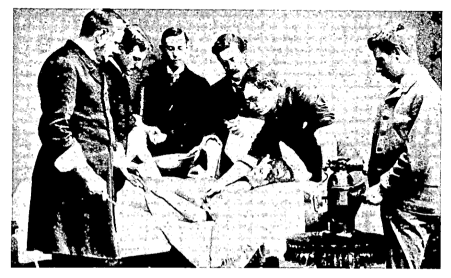

Operation in Aberdeen about 1880. A steam carbolic spray is on the side table.

Cures

All these discoveries revolutionised the art of surgery and facilitated the prevention of disease: but there remained the problem of curing a patient who was already ill. Drugs based on herbs and plants continued to be used to alleviate symptoms, but had little effect on the germ causing the disease. What was needed were chemicals that would attack germs in the body without harming the patient. At the end of the nineteenth century a German scientist, Paul Ehrlich, made a major breakthrough in this area.

It was already known that certain dyes were useful for staining animal tissue prior to examination under a microscope, and Koch had discovered that some dyes actually sought out the bacteria. It was the action and effect of chemicals, particularly chemical dyes being developed for use in the new huge textile industry, which interested Ehrlich. In 1890 he joined Koch's research team in Berlin, and began working on 'magic bullets' which would attack invading germs without harming the body's cells. In 1906 he began working on an arsenic compound as a possible cure for syphilis, and with his assistant, the Japanese Sahachiro Hata, finally located the compound Salvarsan 606. A cure had at last been found, and the groundwork laid for the development of further 'magic bullets'.

Public health and social change

For the medical advances achieved in the nineteenth century to have effect in improving health, there had also to be a fundamental change in the attitudes and responsibilities of society. At the beginning of the nineteenth century disease and a short life expectancy were still regarded as normal, and it was accepted that outbreaks of epidemics of disease would occur from time to time. Although sanitation and an adequate water supply had long been a problem in the big towns, by 1800 conditions in Britain worsened with the influx of people to the industrial towns in the North and the Midlands. People were crowded into old or hastily built accommodation in streets and courtyards near factories in the centre of towns. Whole neighbourhoods were built where there was no water or sanitation. As a result thousands of people died every year from tuberculosis, typhus and typhoid.

So long as people were unaware of the connection between dirt and disease, conditions did not improve. Moreover, even when the cause of disease became evident there existed no legislative body responsible for organising a proper system of sanitation that could implement change. The *laissez faire* attitude of the British government did not permit it to interfere, and it was left up to town councils to make their own arrangements.

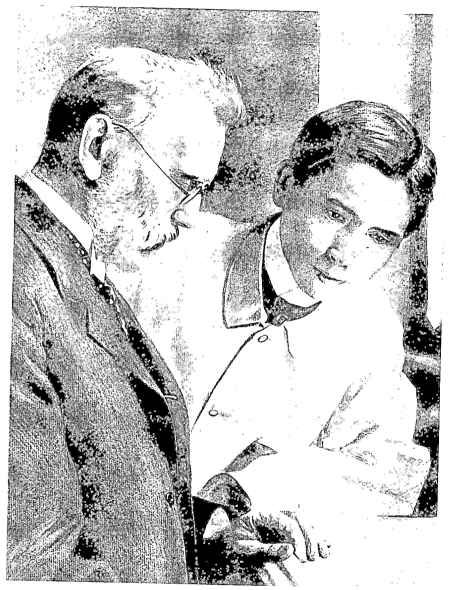

Paul Ehrlich, the German scientist, with his assistant, Sahachiro Hata; they discovered a cure for syphilis.

In the late eighteenth century there had been attempts to improve sanitary conditions in some parts of Britain, where drains might be covered and sewers improved. A mains water system was unknown and cesspools were in use in London as late as the mid-nineteenth century. In

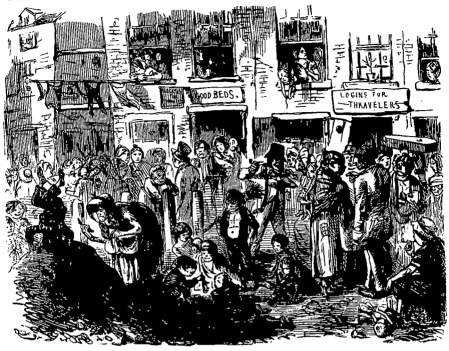

A COURT FOR KING CHOLERA.

Cartoon showing the terrible conditions in cities which encouraged the spread of cholera. (Punch, *25 September 1852*)

1831 an outbreak of cholera swept Britain. The ravages caused by the epidemic were so great that no-one could ignore the disease or the fact that it most affected overcrowded areas of towns. Fear of the disease instigated a concern for public health, but such concern dissipated as the outbreak receded, and improvements in sanitation were piecemeal.

Another outbreak of cholera, and the publication of Edwin Chadwick's *Report on the Sanitary Condition of the Labouring Population of Great Britain* in 1842 describing the dreadful living conditions of masses of people, led to the passing of the Public Health Act in 1848. It took a third outbreak of cholera in 1865, however, finally to convince the most stalwart opponents of public health schemes that legislation was necessary. Yet housing remained appalling, the death rate among children was very high, and better water and sanitation did not improve the general health of adults in poor families. The outbreak of the Boer War in 1899 revealed that 40 per cent of volunteers were medically unfit. Better homes, food, and adequate clothing and medical help for mothers and young children were needed. As the twentieth century dawned, it was beginning to be realised that health and welfare of the public should be one of the country's most important concerns.

THE TWENTIETH CENTURY

We stand on the threshold of an age which is to herald the
recognition of the mother and her child, to give public health work
that human touch it has hitherto lacked, and to modify those glaring
inequalities in social life and conditions which are destructive alike
of infancy and the ideals of Christian citizenship.
*Speech by the Chairman of the Bradford Health Committee at the
opening of the Municipal Maternity Home, 15 March 1915.*

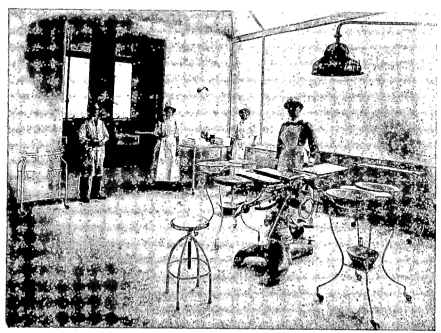

The operating theatre in Kings College Hospital, April 1914.

127

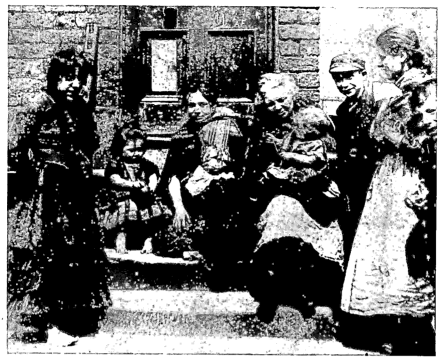

A group of working women and their children, Liverpool, 1895.

THE EARLY YEARS

> The State has to realise that if it wants citizens, and healthy citizens,
> it must make it possible for men and women to have families while
> having a full life themselves, and giving a full life to their children.[1]

By the close of the nineteenth century, a number of major medical
milestones had been reached and passed. In terms of what medicine had
to offer her, the parturient woman was considerably better off than she
had been only fifty years before. And in case of ultimate need, the door to
Caesarean birth had been opened.

The speciality of obstetrics, however, was still in its infancy, and there
were major areas waiting for exploration, many problems still to be
solved. The most important — and it was to be some fifty years more
before significant steps were to be taken — was in the achievement of a
substantial reduction of maternal and perinatal mortality.

In Britain at the turn of the century, a concern for the low birth rate and
the general health and robustness of babies and children had begun to
prompt politicians and pressure groups — particularly the increasingly
influential and vocal women's groups — to turn the attention of the

nation towards infant and maternal welfare. Following concern around the time of the Boer War when it was noticed that the strength and efficiency of British troops left a great deal to be desired, the Interdepartmental Committee on the Physical Deterioration of the Population was appointed and a report was published in 1904. It acknowledged that it was in the nation's interests to safeguard the next generation and improve the race.[2] Soon after followed the Relief (School Children) Order, 1905; the Education (Provision of Meals) Act, 1906, which provided school meals for the needy; and the Education (Administrative Provisions) Act 1907, providing medical inspections in the schools.

George Newman, Chief Medical Officer to the Ministry of Health, in an Annual Report to the Board of Education in 1913 acknowledged that 'the health of the nation is dependent on the health of the child', and 'the health of the child is dependent on the health of the infant and its mother'.[3]

Women were pressurised — by a sector of the population which was plainly reacting against the militant suffragist movement which was so strong in the early years of the century — not to take paid employment outside the home, but to stay and look after their children. Early moves towards state concern for health were backed up by the establishment of 'milk depots' in various parts of Britain; the aim of these depots was to

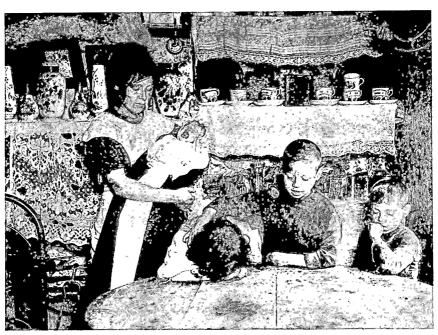

The cruelty of poverty, London, 1912.

reduce the risk of infant mortality from infected milk by supplying municipal control over the milk from cow to baby. The health and progress of the baby were then monitored.

In addition, home visiting had begun as early as 1860, and health visitors were not uncommon by the turn of the century. The 1907 Notification of Births Act required that the local Medical Officer of Health be informed as soon as possible after the birth of a baby. He could then arrange for a health visitor to call on the mother and baby. By 1910 there existed at least 3,000 health visitors. The home visiting network, in tandem with the milk depots and the monitoring of infant progress, could be viewed in two ways: they showed on the one hand the beginnings of a national concern for health and welfare that was the precursor of the setting up of the National Health Service in 1947-48, and on the other hand they represented an intrusion into the whole area of motherhood by an ever-growing army of professionals — medical men, health care administrators, the government. Education of mothers — even of girls of school age — in the art of housekeeping and motherhood, was set into full swing.

Early concern for the health of the nation's young was followed by the traumatic effect of loss of life in the First World War and, as a result, there was an increasing intervention by the state in welfare matters.

The problems of perinatal and maternal mortality, however, were

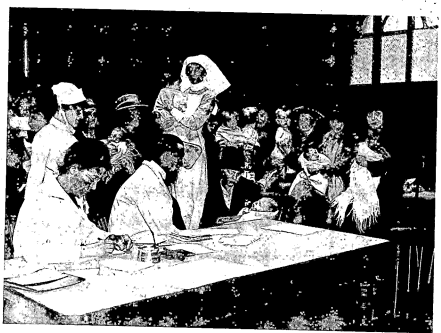

The Children's Department, St Thomas's Hospital, 1921.

largely regarded as clinical ones, and this was a view reinforced by the emerging breed of obstetricians, no longer mere man midwives, but specialists with a rapidly increasing store of medical knowledge at their disposal. The emphasis moved, increasingly, to the clinical and technological problems associated with birth, all too often to the exclusion of social or economic factors which might lie behind the mortality statistics. Hospital care of labour and birth became inevitable as medical innovations demanded a higher standard of knowledge and competence; if these advances were to be applied and administered, then doctors were going to become ever more involved.

Welfare and mortality

While the emphasis on birth itself began to swing towards medicine, enlightened officials realised that many of the causes of infant and neonatal mortality were social and economic, and turned their attention to improved welfare; but it was not until the First World War that a link between fetal and neonatal deaths and maternal welfare was recognised, and attention was extended to antenatal care.

Many welfare schemes were hampered by attitudes to poverty and state interference. There were those, of course, who argued that it was the 'unfit' who died anyway, and that to preserve their lives would weaken the race. Grants and benefits were looked on suspiciously — many people were too proud to accept what they saw as 'charity'. In addition, 'responsibility for the care of women and children was assumed to rest in the hands of a male provider'.[4] Thus, when National Health Insurance was introduced in 1911, it provided only a one-off maternity payment for pregnant mothers, and no other form of insurance. It took some considerable time for the Victorian 'self-help' attitude — designed to make the idea of work more attractive than any form of state assistance — to give way to a new acceptance of state responsibility for welfare.

Slowly official bodies, and writers on the subject, began to recommend that the mother take care of her own health.[5] J W Ballantyne, originator of the notion of antenatal care, made no mention of the mother's health in his 1904 text,[6] but vocal in their insistence on the care of the mother were the women's groups of the period. In 1917, the Women's Co-operative Guild demanded that 'the care of the mother should have equal consideration with the care of the infant'.[7]

By the 1920s, attention to the welfare of mothers had become something of a necessity. Tuberculosis might be the largest cause of death, but death in childbirth claimed 17 per cent of all women's lives during this period. Having a baby was still a terrifyingly dangerous experience.

This left the politicians with a dilemma. With the birth rate falling, there was a pressing need to increase it — but how could they encourage women to have more children when it was so obviously dangerous? And this at a time when women were at last beginning to gain some control over *when* they wanted to have a child.

Two points were apparent: welfare services should be improved, and maternal mortality reduced. Dr Janet Campbell, Senior Medical Officer to the Ministry of Health, recognised the problem, and was the author of the first Government Report on maternal mortality in 1924. Her report pinpointed various problems, in particular long-term maternal ill-health as a consequence of child bearing and a great 'burden of avoidable suffering'.[8] She singled out five major areas requiring attention: sanitation and housing, the employment of women, rickets — causing difficult delivery, abortion or miscarriage (leading to sepsis) — and, first and foremost, the quality of professional attendance, antenatally, at delivery and postnatally.

This government report was the tip of an iceberg insofar as the subject of maternal deaths was concerned. Pressure to improve the situation was great, and widespread.

Certainly this was not an issue that women were going to allow to be dropped quietly. In 1930 Sylvia Pankhurst, daughter of the famous Emmeline, and herself an ardent feminist wrote a book called *Save the Mothers*, in which she deplored the 'contemptuous neglect of the mother's needs and her all-important function',[9] and proposed a 'national maternity service' with wide-ranging measures such as employment protection and social as well as antenatal care.

In 1927 an unofficial pressure group, the Maternal Mortality Committee, was formed for the specific purpose of lobbying Parliament on the issue. In 1932 the group made much of a Government report which stated that 45.9 per cent of deaths investigated were due to a 'primary avoidable factor' — in other words, they could have been prevented.[10] The news that such a very high proportion of deaths need not have happened was not designed to support the image of a caring government, though in response the Government continued to try to reassure women as to the relative safety of childbirth.[11] Doctors, keen to cover up any shortcomings within the profession, advocated that maternal mortality was a matter for internal study rather than public debate; and the popular women's magazines, which have always had a tendency to regard birth and motherhood through rose-coloured glasses, swept the issue adroitly to one side.

Since the 1950s, there have been many studies of the cumulative effects of social status, environment and biological factors on the deaths of infants and mothers, as well as investigations of the more obvious medical factors affecting death. In the 1920s and 30s, however, these

. effects were more or less ignored. Now it is recognised that social grouping, height and obstetric history all have an influence on performance in labour and birth. Working-class women tend to live in poorer areas, marry younger, and bear more children. Environment — not necessarily in the immediate past, but back through a generation or more has proved to be critical: 'women are still paying the price of our early and rapid industrial development'.[12]

Glasgow provided a classic example of the sort of conditions which researchers now know to be detrimental:

> The City of Glasgow, and the whole of Clydeside, which contained 60 per cent of Scotland's population, helped to pioneer the industrial expansion of the 19th century and became one of the places where 'wealth accumulates and men decay'. Many of the inhabitants of Glasgow lived in degradation, crowded together in tenement slums. Few of the slum children after weaning drank milk, except in the smallest quantities. Smoke from the factories and the domestic coal fires shut out the sun. Rickets was so common that Glasgow surgeons became famous for their skill in performing osteotomy to straighten crooked legs. . . . Glasgow surgeons were the first to perform Caesarean section successfully for obstructed labour due to rachitic deformity of the pelvis.[13]

For one student maternity nurse in Glasgow in the 1930s, recreation took a particular form:

> . . . we would eye the female population as they passed, picking out a specimen here, another there, for individual comment. It wasn't their pretty faces or smart rig-outs that intrigued us, it was their torsos and lower limbs, for Glasgow in those days boasted some of the finest specimens in the country.[14]

The effect on childbearing women of deficiencies caused by rickets, a direct result of a poor environment, was painfully obvious. Other social and environmental conditions, particularly poor nutrition were, at the time, all too often ignored.

The heavy toll taken of health by the repeated cycle of pregnancy, sickness and poverty was clearly shown by Margaret Llewelyn Davies in her book, *Maternity: Letters from Working Women*, published in 1915. This series of letters, collected in response to a questionnaire sent out to wives of working men, presents a heartrending picture of what life was like for the working-class mother in the early years of the century. Ignorance is confessed everywhere; and a modesty and embarrassment so marked that in very many cases no doctor was consulted during pregnancy-related illnesses except at the last extremity. Poverty was often dire, particularly when families were very large and income fluctuated because of seasonal work or illness. Many women confessed that their husbands drank away their income; others found that they got through only with the help and support of their husbands. Malnutrition, particularly lack of nourishment during pregnancy, was given as the cause of many stillbirths, weak infants or feeble mothers who were unable to cope with the day to day chores of running the home after the birth. Many mothers miscarried after undertaking strenuous domestic chores — lifting the wash tub or doing heavy domestic cleaning.

Despite pressure from a sector of society which felt that 'a woman's place was in the home', there was no evidence to suggest that industrial employment affected infant or maternal mortality. Indeed, it seemed from evidence accumulated during the First World War about women who worked in munitions factories that such work had a beneficial effect on the mortality figures. Much more damaging were domestic chores:

> Outside employment is often less arduous than much of the household work ordinarily done by the mother of a family, and relief when necessary from heavy housework seems of greater practical importance than the restriction of paid employment.[15]

The social conditions of the time, particularly among the poor, clearly demanded improvement.

No wonder, then, that in her introduction to her book, Margaret Llewelyn Davies pressed for greater responsibility by the state:

> The State first has to realise that if it wants citizens, and healthy citizens, it must make it possible for men and women to have families while living full lives themselves, and giving a full life to their children. . . . The first requisite is the improvement of the economic position of the family. . . . It should be noted that the essence of the Guild scheme is that municipal, not philanthropic, action is wanted. It is not charity, but the united action of the community of citizens which will remove a widespread social evil. The community is performing a duty, not bestowing a charity, in providing itself with the bare necessities for tolerable existence.[16]

The women who wrote to Margaret Davies — the survivors — had had a very high number of live births and a considerable number of stillbirths and miscarriages. They seemed to be plagued at least by very minor, if not major, ailments — constipation, varicose veins, poor teeth, internal wounds from previous births. Inquiries in 1939 by the Women's Health Inquiry Committee turned up similarly common health problems, and there was a pressing concern about morbidity as well as mortality. Pressure took effect in the shape of the establishment of a Ministry of Health in 1919, with Janet Campbell as Senior Medical Officer to the Maternity and Child Welfare Section. Campbell was instrumental in persuading the Ministry to set up the 1928 Departmental Committee on Maternal Mortality and Morbidity, of which she was a member. The Committee was chaired by George Newman, Chief Medical Officer to the

Ministry of Health. The Committee attempted to reconcile the conflicting evidence of, on the one hand, the medical profession, which claimed that high mortality rates were the result of poor environment; and, on the other, lay organisations and pressure groups which claimed that the fault lay with the low standards of clinical care. Medical opinion remained firm in the belief that ignorance and unwillingness to co-operate on behalf of mothers was the primary cause of mortality:

> The patient herself is often her own worst enemy, whether from ignorance or apathy, illhealth or prejudice, etc, and until she is able and willing to co-operate doctors' and nurses' attempts to assist her can never be fully effective.[17]

Non attendance at antenatal clinics is, in the opinion of antenatal care supporters, still a major cause of morbidity. Yet by the 1930s there was no evidence that antenatal care was reducing mortality in childbirth. Regarding an inquiry, George Newman, for his part, felt that such a move would be both expensive and undesirable — the results would be too embarrassing. In a document addressed to the Secretary of State and dated 26 October 1932 he wrote,

> Childbirth has always been woman's travail, and always will be . . . the broad fact remains, first that childbirth is a heavy strain on the physique of any woman and the bodies of many must therefore be impaired, secondly, that there is in modern civilised nations an insufficient number of organised facilities for effective treatment.[18]

The problem being too big to tackle, it seemed that women would just have to go on suffering regardless.

The American concern for health

In America, the campaign for healthier children began roughly at the same time as it did in Britain. In the late years of the nineteenth century, the American middle classes began to limit their families through the use of birth control, and they began to expect a better quality of health than they had hitherto enjoyed. Motherhood began to be 'professionalised'[19] — a trait paralleled in Britain by the vocal women's groups who, by pressing for more and more help for the mother, hoped to raise the status of women at home in the eyes of society. Magazines, books and articles proliferated on the subject of parenthood, elevating it from a 'natural' to a 'scientific' matter. In America, as in Britain, the concern for child health led to an examination of birth practices rather than maternal care, although it was plain that by the turn of the century women who worked long hours in the big industrial factories suffered more ill health and more infant deaths than their better fed middle-class counterparts.

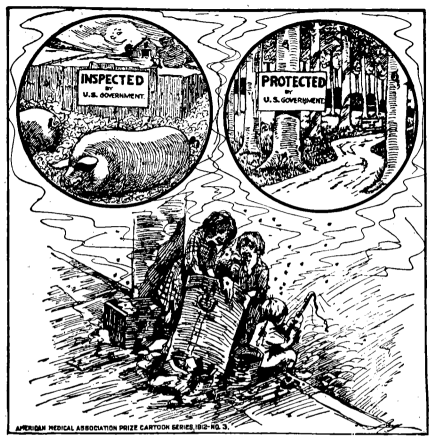

The irony of legislation – or the lack of it – is captured in this 1920 cartoon.

In 1904 the National Child Labor Committee was formed to promote the formation of a national children's bureau to look at child welfare and to collect statistics about infant mortality. Their proposals were not finally realised until 1912, when at last a Children's Bureau was set up. Julia Lathrop, appointed to its head, made one of her first tasks the gathering of reliable statistics about birth and death; and one by one the states passed acts to enforce registration of these events. At the end of the 1920s, for the first time, it was possible to examine statistics to ascertain mortality in mothers and babies. The results were not good. America, it appeared, did not compare favourably with other western industrialised nations.

Other studies introduced by the Bureau revealed another striking fact —the higher the family income, the better were the chances of infant survival. Possibly there was an effect on poorer families of long working hours spent by the mother during pregnancy. Postnatally, it was thought that poorly sterilised feeding bottles of those mothers forced to return to work, and therefore unable to breastfeed, was an important contributory factor to infant diarrhoea, a major cause of death. As in Britain, an educational campaign was launched.

Prenatal care began to be regarded as a means of reducing complications during birth; but it was also clear that the majority of the urban poor had no prenatal care at all. The rural poor — even sometimes the rural middle classes — were even worse off. In the huge American countryside, the effects of isolation were telling. It was all too common for no doctor or trained attendant to be present at the delivery. The cost of medical aid, or the distance from such aid, prevented many people from getting the care they needed during pregnancy and birth.

Appalled by what she discovered, Lathrop proposed a Bill 'for the protection of maternity and infancy', outlining maternity care as a woman's right regardless of income, and not as a charity. The Bill died in its committee stage.

War, as ever, brought changes in needs and enforced changes in attitude. The *Ladies' Home Journal* printed a plea for the reduction of mortality rates:

> During the nineteen months we were at war, for every soldier who died as a result of wounds, one mother in the United States went down into the valley of the shadow and did not return.[20]

The comparison may have been exaggerated, but the message got home. In 1919 Senator Morris Sheppard and Representative Horace Mann Towner had reintroduced Lathrop's measure. It met with considerable opposition. The proposal for a national health service had been rejected as 'a socialistic scheme unsuited to American government', and the American Medical Association orchestrated aggressive opposition to this measure also. But support was strong — very strong — and finally it was the achievement of women's suffrage that forced the Bill through. Twenty million voters could not be ignored.

The money granted by the Sheppard-Towner Act lasted from 1921-29, during which time there was considerable evidence that through prenatal care and supervision, maternal death from eclampsia had fallen dramatically. But in 1929 the money came to an end, and was not to be reintroduced until 1935 under the Social Security Act.

The medical factor

In Britain, despite slow beginnings in improvements in social conditions, the maternal mortality rate showed no sign of decline in the 1920s and 30s. Official reports, as earlier, concentrated on the medical and clinical reasons for death. But even so, reasons for death could be complex and difficult to pinpoint. The three main stages of childbirth — antenatal, labour and postnatal — normally involved attendance by at least three different people; thus defining the cause of death and attributing blame was no easy task.

By this period, many individuals and institutions were involved in overseeing the birth process — consultants in specialist hospitals, GPs, independent and institutional midwives and local authority clinics. When, finally, the Committee on Maternal Mortality and Morbidity was appointed in 1929, the hospitals under consultant obstetricians dominated the process of delivery. The Committee's investigations looked at the immediate causes of death — and the opinion of specialists in the medical profession was considered desirable. Attention was therefore directed to *abnormal* pregnancy and labour.

As a result, pregnancy came to be regarded increasingly as an illness, and it was treated as such. Birth became more and more clinicalised. Obstetricians and committees began to stress the importance of their own particular techniques — that is, techniques of labour management that had been developed to some extent for hospital convenience. Local authority clinics, too, strove for a more 'scientific' approach to the kind of care they provided.

Obstetrics was still a relatively new speciality in medicine. Although a chair in midwifery had been established in Edinburgh as early as 1726, there were few comparable posts elsewhere until the interwar period of the twentieth century. Most of the training of midwives and doctors in the management of labour was obtained in the districts. Public concern about the problem of maternal deaths brought a new focus on the whole area of obstetrics. Recognition came at last for specialists in the field, and in 1929 the British College of Obstetricians and Gynaecologists was formed. (It achieved the accolade 'Royal' in 1938.) The main aim of the College was to establish a standard of training and examination in the field.

It was abundantly clear to both doctors and women alike that the main causes of death at this time were sepsis and haemorrhage. Both hazards, it seemed, could be treated more effectively in hospital than at home. Women, therefore, tended to go along with the recommendations of the Ministry of Health regarding the necessity of the presence of a doctor, the need for hospitalisation, for anaesthesia, analgesia (pain relief), episiotomy or forceps.

Yet, ironically, carelessness by some members of the medical profession in personal hygiene and antiseptic routines undoubtedly contributed to continued outbreaks of puerperal fever, and made hospitals potentially extremely hazardous places to be. And the opportunity for bacteria to enter the bloodstream was greatly increased by interventionist techniques. High- and mid-forceps operations, induced labour, version and Caesarean sections all gave bacteria already present in the body the chance to grow, even though the operating environment was aseptic.

Certainly new techniques for the prevention of eclampsia, and for the transfusion of blood, gave the hospital important advantages as a place for delivery, while the growing knowledge of and expertise in the administration of analgesia provided another very great attraction for many women in the first few decades of this century. And finally, and of major importance, new possibilities in the field of obstetric surgery swung the balance. The march to the hospitals had begun.

The Move to the Hospitals

Birth technology was growing and, in Britain, middle-class women supported the trend away from childbirth in the home. They saw specialist care as desirable and recognised that the hospital consultant's knowledge was superior to that of the midwife. They were influenced, too, by their wish for analgesia. At home, midwives were not permitted to administer painkilling drugs, and even doctors, if they were called in, could not give a full anaesthetic. In view of the slowing down of the birth rate — seen in part as fear of the birth process — it was felt to be desirable to remove this fear as much as possible. The plea for analgesia was sympathetically received.

For working-class women, however, hospital was not always a possibility. If there were other small children at home, someone had to look after them. Husbands, struggling to earn a living, were not available for this kind of support, nor was care of small children in their tradition. The Women's Co-operative Guild in 1917 stressed: 'In the opinion of working women themselves one of their most pressing wants is for reliable help in the home ... during confinements.'[21] The need for home helps was recognised in all quarters, but wages were poor and suitable workers difficult to find. Home helping was anything but an attractive career, and was not looked on with great favour by local authorities, who allocated the service very little money in their budgets. In addition, the duties of a home help were rigorously defined; for example, she might wash, but might not mend or darn. For poor women, the age-old tradition of arrangements with neighbours remained in favour.

Some of the letters published in Margaret Llewelyn Davies' book *Maternity* highlighted the problem at its worst:

> For many of my children I have not been able to pay a nurse to look after me, and I have got out of bed on the third day to make my own gruel and fainted away.[22]

I had to depend on my neighbours for what help they could give during labour and the lying-in period. They did their best, but from the second day I had to have my other child with me, undress him and see to all his wants, and was often left six hours without a bite of food. When I got up after ten days my life was a perfect burden to me. I lost my milk and ultimately lost my baby.[23]

For such women hospital was not an option, only a place to be taken in extremity. Yet home was certainly not an attractive alternative:

You find a bed which has been slept on by the husband, wife and one or two children; it has frequently been soaked with urine, the sheets are dirty, and the patient's garments soiled; she has not had a bath. Instead of sterile dressings you have a few old rags or the discharges are allowed to soak into the nightdress which is not changed for days.[24]

Life as a district midwife in the Glasgow slums in the twenties gave one trainee, Mary Thomson, all the experience she could have wished for — and more:

My first call took me to a vermin infested building where babies slept side by side with dogs, cats, rats, bugs, fleas and lice ... I was ushered into a room about five feet square. The patient lay on a bed built into a recess in the wall, and a line of washing — under which I had to duck — spread itself across the room. Two dogs, a tall skinny specimen of the whippet breed and a terrier of uncertain parentage, occupied the space in front of the fire. A large tom cat was draped over the best chair, the only other chair having a hole through the seat of it. The room smelt strongly of soapsuds, bad fish, cat and dog, and the washing dribbled over the floor where little rivulets were cleaning a way through surrounding dirt ...[25]

In Glasgow, city of poverty, every maternity nurse 'on the district' knew that sooner or later she would have to make at least one trip into a house so bug-ridden that it defied contemplation. Mary Thomson made one such trip in the early hours of the morning on a warm summer's day:

I went forward to the bed and turned down the grubby blanket round her, then jumped back into the room with a cry of astonishment. Scattering in all directions as the light caught them, were hundreds of brown insects. They were running all over Lily's half-naked body, under pillows, and into every crevice that would shield them from the light ...

I spent four hours in that crawling, festering room before Lily's son was born ... but at last the baby was born, bathed, dressed, and the question arose as to where I was going to put him. I was horrified by the thought of him being laid in the bed beside his mother and the bugs, but evidently, that was just where he had to go. 'The bugs'll no dae him ony harm,' said his loving grandma. 'He'll have tae get used tae them like the rest o' us.'[26]

Ignorance regarding basic hygiene, as much as poverty, was often the reason for insanitary conditions in very poor homes:

> Cleanliness has made rapid strides since my confinement, for never once can I remember having anything but face, neck and hands washed until I could do things myself, and it was thought certain death to change the underclothes under a week. For a whole week we were obliged to lie on clothes stiff and stained, and the stench under the clothes was abominable, and added to this we were commanded to keep the babies under the clothes.[27]

At the same time, the 'necessities' for a confinement as listed in *The Motherhood Book* of 1934 would have been well beyond the financial means of the average working-class family. Here improvisation was called for; brown paper and newspapers were used instead of rubber sheets and more newspapers for the swabs instead of bowls. In Birmingham in the late 1920s it was reported that one street had a communal 'midwife's bowl and jug' which was passed up and down the street when needed. In rural Oxfordshire, some forty years earlier (where, despite great poverty, cleanliness was regarded as all-imporant), Flora Thomson, author of the classic *Lark Rise to Candleford* described the same kind of communal self-help:

> THE BOX ... appeared simultaneously with every new baby. ... It contained half a dozen of everything — tiny shirts, swathes, long flannel barrows, nighties, and napkins made, and kept in repair, and lent for every confinement by the clergyman's daughter.[28]

In the 1930s, many working-class women felt that 'maternity bags' provided by some local authorities, and containing all the necessities for labour and delivery, were 'charity', and they did not like having to resort to their use. In consequence, although the Women's Co-operative Guild and Women's Labour League demanded that more bags be provided, they were not widely used.

Labour and delivery for the better-off mothers in the early years of the century were a different matter. They, too, were likely to have their babies at home, but they would have a living-in nurse for at least a month. 'Lying-in' was therefore less of a problem — and of course, the conditions in these homes would be considerably more pleasant than those in the poor working-class houses.

One renowned obstetrician, Sir Dugald Baird, was able to maintain that the drop in perinatal and maternal mortality was linked to the rise in hospital deliveries, and at the same time to enjoy the birth of his own four children — at home; and 'made more comfortable and enjoyable for all concerned by the presence of a cook, housemaid, and resident midwife'.[29]

Around the late 1920s and early 30s, private nursing homes began to open — often just converted houses — and it became fashionable for the

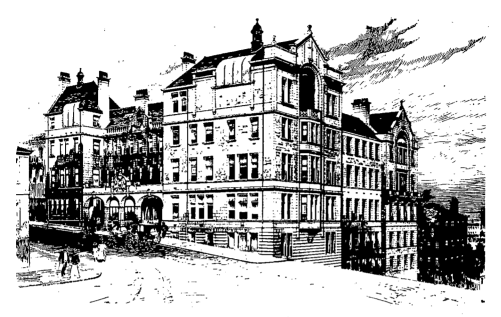

The architect's drawing of the new maternity hospital 'Rottenrow' in Glasgow, built in the early twentieth century.

better-off to have their babies there. If complications developed, the mother would be transferred to a nearby hospital which would have better equipment.

The hospitals before 1930

Between the wars, the number of available hospital beds in Britain rose steadily. In 1920 around 5 per cent of births were thought to require hospitalisation; by 1944 the Royal College of Obstetricians and Gynaecologists felt that provision should be made for the hospitalisation of 70 per cent of all births.[30] In some areas small maternity hospitals were established — some having only GP units and no consultant units — but the trend was for larger units with sixty to seventy beds based in large teaching hospitals.

Once arrangements had been made to provide such large units, it became necessary to maintain their quota of patients. University College Hospital in London increased its number of beds 'to comply with demand'; but it also made cuts in the number of district midwives available, so that mothers had little alternative but to come into hospital. With the emphasis swinging from home to hospital, many students were trained to deal with emergencies under hospital conditions alone.

143

Obstetricians, co-opted increasingly to panels and committees, recommended growth in hospitalisation; but not all hospitals were equipped to cope with increased numbers of parturient women. In 1929 under the Local Government Act the local authorities took control of Poor Law institutions. Such institutions were not designed for maternity care. In the Elizabeth Garrett Anderson Hospital there was no separate labour ward before 1929, and conditions were decidedly overcrowded. Lambeth was dirty and had obsolete bathroom facilities; and at St Pancras in 1936 there were still no proper sterilisers, no isolation ward for cases of sepsis. When the London County Council permitted any mother who wished to attend hospital for delivery, overcrowding problems grew still further.

Attention to aseptic procedures was put forward as one of the main virtues of hospital birth — and indeed, in comparison with the distressing conditions of dirt and deprivation in the homes of the very poor, such attractions might have seemed a great advantage. In stressed, pressured conditions, however, basic procedures were often overlooked. In middle-class nursing homes, a reported case of sepsis could warrant the temporary closure of the entire institution. To avoid this, many cases were not isolated, or not reported. Other hospitals, of course, had excellent records — and correspondingly low mortality statistics.

Big teaching hospitals such as Glasgow's Royal Maternity Hospital normally had stringent procedures:

> If a puerperal patient develops a rise of temperature, she may be heading for anything from housemaid's knee to deadly septicemia. In those pre-antibiotic days, a rise of temperature above a hundred degrees in a postnatal ward was likely to disorganise the whole construction of life in a ward . . . If a second patient developed a rise in temperature in the wake of the first one, the whole senior staff went mad. The ward would be cleared, fumigated, scraped, scrubbed and carbolised until every germ for miles beat a hasty retreat.[31]

In the United States, hospitalisation became more widespread earlier than in Britain. After the introduction of the Sheppard-Towner Act in 1921, middle-class women took it upon themselves to search for the best care that they could afford. Hospitals advertised themselves as being 'germ free' and 'sterile', and birth in hospital meant that the messiness involved in the birth process could be kept out of the home — important in an age where new mechanical household aids enabled even the poorer middle-class wife with no domestic help to be 'houseproud'.

Hospitals advertised 'trained attendance day and night', and in addition there was a wide variety of medical equipment available in the hospitals — X-ray machines, laboratories, and so on. New technology and new operative skills were available for infants in danger; and on top of it all, there was someone to wait on you day and night, feed you, wash you, and take the care of running the home off your shoulders. New hospitals were built that were charming, fresh, home-like in appearance, but with all mod cons — telephones, buzzers, rooms provided for the use of husbands.

The cost of all this, in a country where there were no insurance schemes, was high. Yet the mass of publicity literature pressed young couples to 'go for the best'. And the best, it was widely assumed, was the most expensive.

By the early 1930s in America, 60-75 per cent of births in many cities took place in hospitals. Costs were increasing all the time, as the number of specialists involved in the birth process increased — surgeons, anaesthetists, consultants, more expensive equipment, more drugs. Despite the candy floss, however, American women did not always get what they thought they were paying for. There existed no training standards for obstetricians, and any general practitioner could at that time perform any obstetric operation, however inexperienced or ill equipped he might be to do so. In 1930 the American Board of Obstetrics and Gynaecology was established, partly with a view to improving training standards.

A report on maternal deaths between 1930 and 1932 concluded that of the 2,401 deaths studied, two-thirds had been avoidable. The report castigated the 'ignorance and insufficient training of the attendant' and

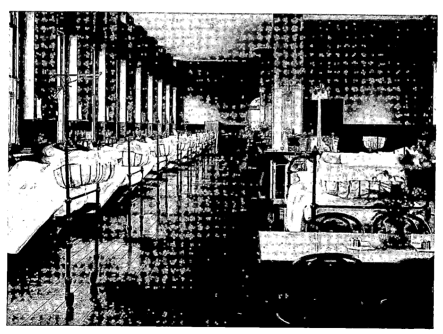

Mary Maternity ward, St Thomas's Hospital, April 1921.

reported on poor standards of asepsis in the hospitals.[32]

Another report published the same year pinpointed the fact that maternal mortality had shown no decline between 1915 and 1930, despite the increase in hospital delivery, antenatal care and aseptic techniques. Deaths of babies from birth injuries in the same period had actually increased.[33] Death was attributed in part to inadequate antenatal care, and in part to the frequent and unnecessary intervention in the labour and birth process, often for quite inadequate reasons, and with insufficient attention to aseptic routines.

Following these reports, training standards were more rigorously applied; unskilled people were forbidden to undertake tasks for which they had no training, and standards of asepsis were more strictly supervised. Between 1936 and 1955 mortality rates dropped markedly. New routines, as well as new antibiotic drugs, accounted for most of the improvement. Intervention, if anything, increased, but it was usually undertaken by qualified staff:

> Birth remained, in the view of the doctors, an abnormal, pathogenic process which required routine medical assistance to prevent disaster. Professional and public concern for safety had pruned away improper techniques and egregious incompetence, but not the philosophy that medical arts created the healthful birth.[34]

It was a philosophy that was to set the tone for the modern age of obstetrics.

The midwife

In America, while doctors gained a grip of the birth process, the status and role of the midwife were decreasing with equal rapidity. Yet even while, strictly speaking, midwifery was illegal as late as 1935 figures from Massachusetts showed that the midwife was alive and practising.

The midwife, ever popular with the immigrant working classes, provided a much more comprehensive service than the doctor. As in earlier times she would not merely attend the birth, but very often would also clean the house, do the laundry and stay with the woman for some days after the birth. Her fees were considerably lower too. In rural Texas in 1930, women, asked why they had called a midwife rather than a doctor, replied:

> Had midwife because could get her for 75 cents, doctor cost $15,

and

> Molly was closer and doctor higher. Did my washing and charged only $5. Really worth more.[35]

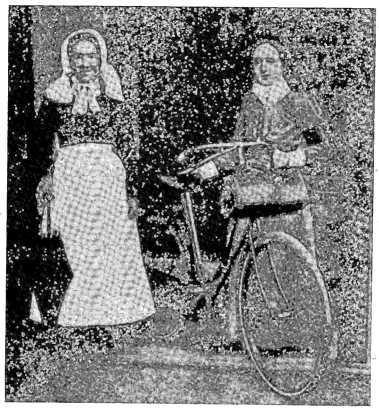

The Midwives' Act of 1902 brought change. The old 'granny midwife' on the left, on the right, the new, smarter, better trained licensed midwife.

In America, particularly among some immigrant races, the tradition of male birth attendants was unthinkable. The midwife provided the only possible alternative with any skill or experience. Yet the picture presented of these immigrant midwives — particularly by parties with a vested interest in diminishing their role — was much akin to that of the 'granny' midwife of history — ignorant, filthy, superstitious, hidebound. Certainly, age-old methods of procuring abortions were not unknown to these women.

The question remained: what to do with the midwife? The situation in the States was quite different from that in Europe. In America by the twentieth century midwifery was synonymous with these so-called ignorant, illiterate immigrant women. There was no question of providing them with adequate training. Nor did the profession of midwife have any status in the eyes of women generally, and thus it was unlikely to attract women of education and respectability to its ranks. Their disappearance was inevitable. It was clear, however, that midwives were not going to disappear overnight. In the meantime, state authorities sought to provide some measure of supervision to ensure cleanliness, to persuade the midwife to call a doctor should any abnormality appear, to administer no drugs, to apply silver nitrate drops after birth (to avoid blindness), and to register the birth.

Gradually, however, second-generation immigrants began to follow American custom and seek out doctors themselves. Few new midwives appeared after the restriction of immigration in 1919, for the rewards were low and there were better-paid jobs to be had. Nevertheless, a new breed of maternity nurse did appear in America in the 1930s — the nurse-midwife. Nurse-midwives grew out of a nursing, rather than a midwifery, tradition. They took their training as public health nurses, then were recruited by special organisations such as the Maternity Center Association of New York for further specialist training in midwifery. Always intended to care for the poor, the nurse-midwife continued as part of the public health system, practising in hospital clinics or rural maternity centres. The total number of these nurses, however, remained small.

In Britain, the story of the midwife ran along lines very different from the tale in America. After years of work, the Midwives' Bill had finally passed into law on 31 July 1902 to enact registration and licensing. It was progress of real long-term importance, for it ensured the survival of the midwife, even if she still had to accept a large amount of medical supervision over her activities. It was not until 1920 that the Central Midwives' Board saw its first midwife member, and 1973 saw the first midwife as Chairman of the Board.

At first, the provisions for training set out by the board were low. A three-month course, it was thought, was all that many women would be able to afford. Gradually, as financial support for women in training began to appear from other sources, the period of training increased in 1937, to two years. Eventually, it became the case that the vast majority of midwives were also fully trained nurses.

The new status of the midwife was a matter of concern for general practitioners. They felt more than ever that their income from midwifery work, though small, would be threatened. More importantly, good obstetric care laid the foundations of family care for the next generation for the GP. Changes in attitude thus came gradually. After the introduction of the 1911 National Insurance Act, which made provision for GP care for poor workers, practitioners felt their income more assured: there was a less pressing need to cling to maternity work. The 1914-18 War, too, made a difference to the situation; many doctors were called to the front, leaving midwives to fill at least that part of their service.

The question of who should pay the midwife was always a tricky one. In

1936 (1937 in Scotland) the problem was finally resolved by the introduction of further legislation providing for payment of a salary to midwives by local authorities. The question of who should pay the doctor was resolved at the same time — again, this was to be the responsibility of the local authority. The solution of one problem may have been the genesis of another: it has been argued that extra payments made to GPs when drugs or instruments were used led to a greater intervention in the birth process — and unnecessary intervention can in itself be the cause of problems.

For some time after the enactment of the Midwives' Bill a number of *bona fide* midwives continued to practise. In the late 1920s Mary Thomson in Glasgow met a real 'granny' midwife:

> Granny Green was a star turn. She had given birth to twenty-three weans of her own, and in her spare time she delivered half the weans in and around the Gorbals district of Glasgow in the days when there was no legislation forbidding the practice. She was ninety two when I met her . . . she had a squint at the table, decorated with forceps, scissors, eye-drops, ligatures, swabs, cord-dressings, hypodermic syringe and kidney tray, and said, 'Ah didn't need awl them plasters.'[36]

Many *bona fide* midwives had experience in plenty, but lacked the formal medical training necessary to pass the midwifery examinations. The rules governing their conduct after the introduction of the Act became very strict. Midwives were liable to random inspection at any time. Clothing and equipment were strictly specified, and rules on disinfecting procedures after contact with sepsis were rigorous. Midwives not complying with the rules were liable to prosecution and suspension — a serious matter for an independent woman on a small income.

Training of midwives increased in length from the initial three months to eighteen months, and only for registered nurses. The question of what the midwife should be taught and which duties she should be allowed to perform was important. Should the midwife be allowed to administer analgesia in the home? In 1936, the British College of Obstetricians decided to allow the administration of gas and air — a disappointing decision for the midwife, for the apparatus was expensive, and few midwives could afford to invest in it. The midwife was in general well liked and trusted within the community, particularly by working-class women. Yet at that time, many women were seeking pain relief and if they could not get it in the home, then they were more likely either to go to a nursing home or hospital to deliver their baby, or to call in the doctor. The British Medical Association (BMA) also favoured the idea of making the GP responsible for all antenatal care, and for deciding whether a particular case could be handled by a midwife.

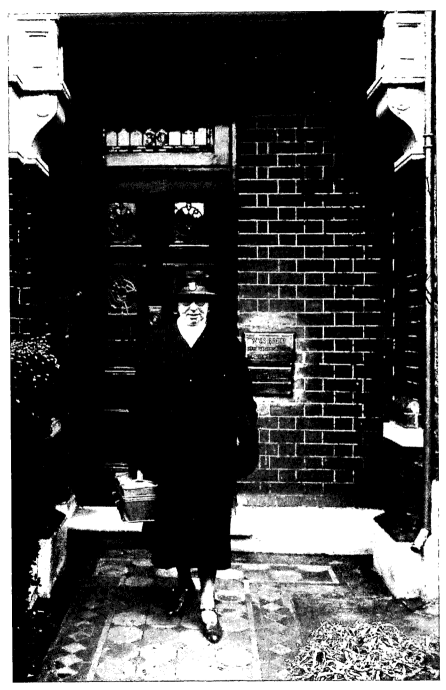

A midwife leaves a call, 1938.

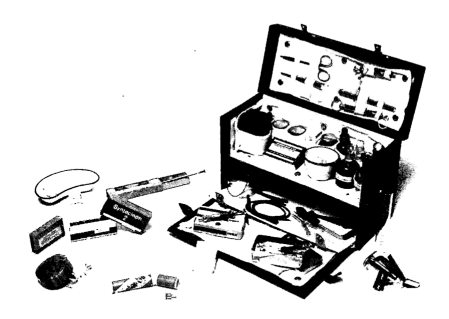

A midwife's bag, used for calls 'on the district'.

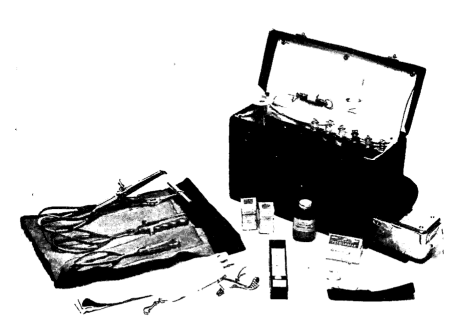

A doctor's bag included his instruments.

The midwife was officially confined, in fact, to the handling of 'normal' birth. Thus legislation had served to accentuate not only the difference in status between medical man and midwife, but

> in the early years of this century, a division thus developed *within* childbearing between the normal and the abnormal.[37]

It was a division which was to have an increasing significance; for the definition of the 'normal' birth was to become one of the areas of dispute in the battle between doctor and midwife for the control of the birth process.

The doctor

Through centuries of tradition, doctors had little or nothing to do with childbirth. Accordingly, the training of doctors in obstetric practice was, in the first two decades of this century, barely adequate. Sir Dugald Baird recalled that in Rottenrow Hospital in Glasgow between 1925 and 1929 he saw few medical students in the wards or antenatal clinics.[38] At University College Hospital in London things were much the same:

> In the twenties there was NO teaching in labour apart from a routine medical school lecture. The plan was for the new list [of obstetric students] to go out with someone of the previous month's list to see a baby born; they were supposed to know all about it . . .[39]

Medical students attending cases on the district were unsupervised. Baird recalled his first encounter with midwifery in his last year as a medical student just after the First World War:

> I had gone out with another student to observe confinements in the home . . . We were called professors — two young professors from the maternity hospital; and I can remember the first one we went to. We opened the door and here was a woman in labour having very strong pains, and we stood there paralysed; we didn't know what to do. And this woman said — I can always remember what she said — 'Holy Mother of God, doctor, can ye no dae something for me?' And I could do absolutely nothing for her.[40]

As late as 1936 the problem of ill-trained doctors still existed. In Rochdale, a maternal mortality committee found that 'the problem of the doctor presented the greatest difficulty. The training he received was lamentably inadequate at most schools, and the average man went into practice with no real experience . . .'[41] Part of the problem, despite the BMA's insistence on the doctor's right to practise midwifery, was that there were simply not enough births for the GP to build up skill and experience. Midwives increasingly undertook straightforward deliveries, so that the GP had no bank of normal births against which to match his experience of abnormal deliveries.

Unfortunately for the mother to whom the GP was called, the doctor could intervene in the birth process where his more practised midwife counterpart either would not or was not permitted to; and for a busy GP with a hundred other calls on his time, there was no question of waiting long hours to allow for spontaneous delivery. After 1909, the drug pituitrin, for example, was often administered to speed up the action of the uterus. Occasionally, the forceful action of the drug would accelerate labour so greatly that it would cause the rupture of the uterus. Yet it came to be used as often as forceps.

The use — or rather abuse — of forceps was one of the more disturbing sides of the GP home delivery story in the 1920s and 30s. Often, all too often, doctors used forceps incompetently, and were ultimately forced to transport their patients with great speed to the nearest hospital as an 'FFO' or 'Failed Forceps Outside'. Many doctors, too impatient to wait for the full dilatation of the cervix, would apply forceps too early; or else they would use forceps when some part other than the head was presenting. In a 1928 study on unsuccessful forceps cases, anxiety and impatience were given as the reason for FFO in approximately one-third of the cases studied.[42] Fatalities from FFOs were high; one in ten mothers died later in hospital and two-thirds of the babies died.

Certainly the performance of GPs reflected in these tales and figures was not designed to inspire confidence. Reference to such stories was commonplace in both the newspapers and medical literature of the day:

> It is a pathetic and humiliating sight to see a healthy young woman dying in childbed, with her little wedding presents as yet untarnished about her, because the medical attendant has thought it right to risk the production of injuries in a first and normal labour.[43]

Compare this with Flora Thomson's notes about rural Oxfordshire around the same period:

> The only cash outlay in an ordinary confinement was half a crown, the fee of the old woman who, as she said, saw the beginning and the end of everybody. She was, of course, not a certified midwife; but she was a decent, kind, intelligent old body, clean in her person and methods and very kind ... complications at birth were rare; but in the two or three cases where they did occur during her practice, old Mrs Quinton had sufficient skill to recognise the symptoms and send post-haste for the doctor. No mother lost her life in childbed during the decade.[44]

When, in 1916, there was an unexpected fall in perinatal mortality, it was conjectured that the drop was due to the paucity of doctors available for general practice because of the war; midwives, to a large extent taking over, did not use forceps or other means of obstetric intervention.[45] By 1929, it seemed that progress was in a backward direction. Henry Jellett complained in that year that doctors were turning 'a physiological process in a healthy woman into a death trap'.[46]

The impatience of GPs who applied forceps too eagerly was not always a selfish one. 'The medical attendant may not find it altogether easy to resist the demands of his patient for speedy relief,' wrote Janet Campbell in 1924.[47] The family, gathered around the bed, might well plead with the doctor to curtail the labour pains of the mother.

It may well be clear to us now that the general practitioner of the 1920s and 30s was seldom suitably qualified or experienced to perform obstetric work; yet at the time it was generally agreed that his superior medical training made his attendance at the birth desirable, particularly where there were complications. It became a method of judging the efficiency and competence of the midwife to ascertain how many times she had called in the doctor. Between 1911 and 1935, the increase of calls on GPs by midwives rose steadily.

Before 1940, neither equipment nor expertise in the hospitals was good enough to make for noticeably greater safety in birth; indeed, the often overcrowded and unhygienic conditions of older hospitals made them decidedly more dangerous. Home remained the normal place of delivery.

During the Second World War, arrangements were made to evacuate pregnant women from areas likely to be bombed, and emergency homes were set up in safer areas — usually in large country houses. These were staffed by midwives and pupil midwives. The arrangement proved most successful, and maternal mortality rates dropped noticeably during this period. Significantly, these homes provided many women with their first experience of institutional birth — and many of them liked the experience. In the view of mothers sent to Lennox Castle in Glasgow 'it was a grand idea because they could get a holiday at the same time'.[48] With birth in institutions rising by as much as 20 or 30 per cent in the early years of the war: '. . . it is probable that the shape of the wartime maternity services was at least a contributory factor in the sharp post-war upturn in the institutional delivery rate.'[49]

Increasing technology has gradually lessened the influence, such as it has been, of the GP on childbirth. It also, finally, disturbed the always delicate balance between the doctor and midwife. In 1959 the Cranbrook Committee concluded that:

> . . . under present day conditions the practice of obstetrics requires the exercise of special skill beyond the competence of general practitioners and a degree of experience that, with the present high institutional confinement rate, the average family doctor is unlikely to be able to maintain.[50]

The post-1930 hospital

Conditions in the homes of the poor in the earlier years of this century could vary from merely cramped to downright filthy. By the 1930s middle-class women had begun a steady drift to the hospitals, which offered a very different kind of birth.

In America the routine became so inflexible that almost every woman would be treated to the same impersonal, often humiliating process. She would be wheeled into the delivery room, rolled onto her back and her feet raised in stirrups — the 'lithotomy' position. Her arms and legs were strapped down so that she was unable to move. Around her was the medical paraphernalia of birth. The treatment would start. Analgesia would be administered, which would demand the administration of oxytocin to speed up the contractions which the analgesic had slowed down. Forceps would be applied, which would necessitate at least local anaesthesia and an episiotomy. The lithotomy position itself would demand the administration of analgesia — and so it would go on.

The mother would not be allowed a companion. She would not be told what was happening to her; nothing would be explained. Stories from American mothers in the 1940s and 50s reflect the way in which the smooth working of the hospital had priority over everything else, the mother's comfort and well-being included:

> When my baby was ready the delivery room wasn't. I was strapped to a table, my legs tied together, so I would 'wait' until a more convenient and 'safer' time to deliver. In the meantime my baby's heartbeat started faltering . . .[51]

Another letter published in the *Ladies' Home Journal* said,

> I was strapped to the delivery room table on Saturday morning and lay there until I was delivered on Sunday afternoon, with the exception of a period early Sunday morning when they needed the delivery table for an unexpected birth.[52]

Again:

> During my second baby's arrival, I was strapped to a table, hands down, knees up. I remember screaming, 'Help me! Help me!' to a nurse who was sitting at a nearby desk. She ignored me. With my third baby, the doctor said at one point, 'Stop your crying at me, I'm not the one who made you pregnant!'[53]

Another mother drew her own conclusions about the reasons for this kind of inhumanity:

> I know of many instances of cruelty, stupidity and harm done to mothers by obstetricians who are callous or completely indifferent to the welfare of their patients. Women are herded like sheep through

> an obstetrical assembly line, are drugged and strapped on tables while their babies are forceps-delivered. Obstetricians today are businessmen who run baby factories. Modern painkillers and methods are used for the convenience of the doctor, not to spare the mother.[54]

In Britain around this time many hospitals, meticulously scrubbed, could present a face as attractive and bright as the most modern of American maternity hospitals. The Glasgow Royal Maternity Hospital in the early 1930s was an inviting place:

> The labour ward was white and spacious, and on that lovely May morning the warm Spring sunshine sparkled through the high curtainless windows and reflected from the smooth painted walls, turning the whole place into a globe of light. The shining mosaic floors, not to be outdone, took up the challenge and sent back glittering sparks of silver and gold into the warm peaceful atmosphere. Rows of spotless handbasins, cream-curtained cubicles, showcases crammed with silver instruments and softly running glass-topped trolleys combined to make this the centre of human interest the most beautiful place in the world. . . . We took our places with mop and pail and proceeded to drench the already spotless floor with boiling water and strong lysol.[55]

However, routines in British hospitals were not nearly as inflexible, nor were interventions as commonplace as in the States. Sir Dugald Baird, practising in Scotland fifty years ago, said:

> . . . in the 1930s, I was doing what young women are advocating now — natural childbirth . . . They could get up and walk around if they wanted to. Then I used to say to them, now what do you want to do? Do you want to push it out yourself, or have it taken out for you? What do you think? — What you did depended on what the patient was like.[56]

Sir Dugald's liberal practice was not the whole story, of course. He himself recalled an occasion when he arrived in Aberdeen:

> . . . going round the lying-in ward I found that about half the women had their knees tied together — and of course they were in bed for about ten days in those days. How would you like to be in bed for ten days with your knees tied together?[57]

Reports of women being left alone in labour, ignorant and fearful, were not uncommon. One woman wrote to obstetrician Dr Grantly Dick Read:

> I was shown into the labour room and left. I began to feel unbearably ill, with severe pains, about 7 o'clock. Nurse had told me not to ring for her, as she could not stay with me . . . I was given medicine at about 10.30 but was not told what it was. What followed afterwards

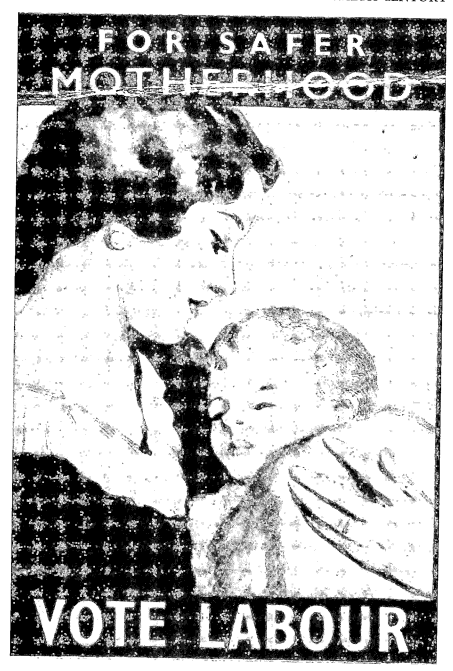

A 1939 political poster promoting maternity care.

was like a ghastly nightmare. I begged the nurse to stop with me, but
she just said the baby would not be born that night, I was to make no
noise, and left me ... One nurse was pulling my arms above my head;
the other was pressing my tummy down ... They buried my head in
pillows to stifle my screams; I thought they would suffocate me ...[58]

Such experiences were to lead to the questioning by women of the whole
nature of the birth experience they were having in hospitals; and Grantly
Dick Read was himself one of those to provoke such questioning. During
the 1930s and 40s, however, the drift to the hospitals continued apace.

The Welfare State and the National Health Service

The move to the hospitals took place amid a growing acceptance that the
state had a responsibility to look after its people. Antenatal care,
beginning to be more common in the 1930s, had established beyond
doubt that poor nutrition was a major cause of both maternal and
neonatal mortality. At the Labour Party Conference in 1934 one speaker
proposed that:

In view of the recent rise in the maternal mortality rate, and the
unchallengeable evidence that one of the contributory causes is the
undernourishment of mothers, this conference calls on HM
Government to arrange for the immediate provision of free milk to
nursing and expectant mothers in necessitous circumstances.[59]

Two years later, John Boyd Orr's *Food, Health and Income* showed
that 10 per cent of the population was unable to afford a minimum diet as
recommended by the British Medical Association, and another 20 per
cent could barely do so. Steps were taken around this time to provide free
milk in schools, but nothing was done for mothers.

Voluntary groups, notably the National Birthday Trust, did distribute
extra foodstuffs at antenatal clinics in certain areas, and the effect on the
death rate appeared to be propitious. The attitude of government,
however, remained unhelpful; it was felt that ignorance about diet and
household management, more than poverty, was at the root of the
problem. It took the outbreak of the Second World War, and renewed
fears about the size and health of the population, for anything concrete to
be done about nutrition, particularly in the shape of free milk schemes. In
June 1940, a National Milk Scheme was introduced, and every pregnant
or nursing mother and every child under five was provided with a daily
free 'pinta', and in addition received free vitamin supplements — fruit
juice, cod-liver oil, rose-hip syrup and vitamin pills.

The low birth rate in the time of war provided a further crisis, and the
government sought a means of encouraging a rise. The question of family
allowance was raised. Finally, in 1942, a proposal was made that a flat rate

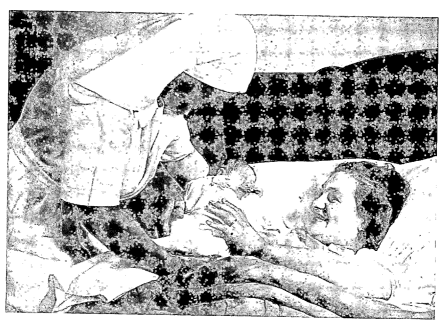

Birth at home, 1946.

allowance of five shillings per week per child should be paid, into the hands of the mother. When the Family Allowances Act was passed in 1945, it gave a payment of five shillings to all children except the first — but, importantly, there was no provision for payment to the mother.

The war had precipitated many crises on the home front; a mass evacuation policy had thrown together people from widely differing backgrounds, and for the first time brought awareness to many of the living conditions of large sectors of the population. In addition, war had fractured the family — fathers were away at the front, mothers out at work, no longer able to care for their children or the aged. There was a gradual but growing acceptance of the need for the state to assume an increasing responsibility for welfare.

Regarding motherhood, however, successive governments refused to accept that poverty was the cause of high infant and maternal mortality rates, preferring to view the cause as one of maternal ignorance. Educational programmes, implemented by health visitors and infant welfare centres, were provided instead of a good basic minimum income. Maternal and infant mortality were treated as medical problems, and made the way in which the birth process itself was handled increasingly 'scientific'.

State acceptance for responsibility of health came slowly. Family Allowance in 1945 — paid to the father — was the first of a number of reforms. Meanwhile, the British Medical Planning Commission

159

published a report in 1942 suggesting that the quality of medical care should be the same for rich and poor. The suggestion was a radical one. It coincided with the publication of the report of the Beveridge Committee on Social and Allied Services, which proposed the abolition of all means tests in health treatment, and free health facilities for everyone. The report was widely acclaimed, although amongst the medical profession there was considerable worry about the administration of the service and methods of payment. Many doctors were concerned as to whether all private practice would disappear. Such questions were resolved gradually, and plans for the National Health Service (NHS) were scheduled for implementation on 5 July 1948.

One immediately noticeable result was that no longer was the midwife the first point of contact for the pregnant woman. That role fell, increasingly, to the GP, while midwives began to work more and more within hospitals and less and less in the community. In addition, the NHS meant that every mother became entitled to free care before, during and after birth, and made the hospitals accessible to all.

From 1927 to 1946, the percentage of women giving birth in a hospital or maternity home increased from 15 to 54 per cent — although the *British Medical Journal* was still able to recommend that 'the proper place for confinement is the patient's own home'.[60] By 1958, that figure had risen to 64 per cent. And the following year the Maternity Services (Cranbrook) Committee of the Ministry of Health made the recommendation that 'provision should be made over the country as a

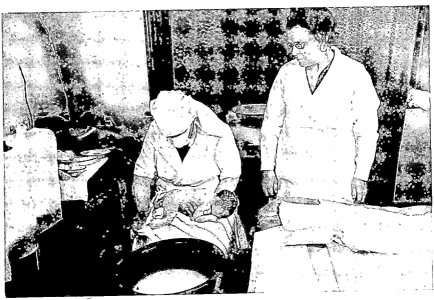

Birth at home, 1946.

whole of a sufficient number of beds to allow an average of 70 per cent institutional confinements.'[61] At last official opinion had shifted in line with the thinking of consultants.

When the Peel Committee reported in 1970,[62] opinion had swung even further in favour of hospitalisation. The greater safety of hospital confinement, it was argued, justified the provision of facilities for all mothers:

> It was unanimously agreed that the upward trend in hospital confinement would continue . . . There seems to be a gradually increasing appreciation in the profession and amongst the general public that confinement in hospital is the safest arrangement, irrespective of considerations of finance or convenience.[63]

One further factor had a critical bearing on the growth of hospital births. During the 1960s, women began to be able to control their fertility more effectively than they ever had before — for this was the age of the pill. Availability of contraception for all women and not just the educated few, combined with the ability of gynaecologists simply and quickly to perform sterilisations, meant that women were able at last to choose to have fewer children. Hospital facilities already in existence could now be used by a larger proportion of women.

By 1974, 95.6 per cent of all babies in Britain were born in a hospital or other institution. From 1946 to 1958 the change of control of the birth process was from private to NHS practice. From 1958, even despite the increase of GP units within hospitals, the hold of consultants was tightening. Cranbrook had recommended that 'a consultant should have overall responsibility of the general practitioner maternity beds'.[64] In 1980 the Short Report on Perinatal and Neonatal Mortality recommended that 'an increasing number of mothers be delivered in large units . . . and that home delivery is phased out further'.[65] Official pressure on women to give birth in the hospital was becoming implacable.

This wholesale hospitalisation had already begun, inevitably, to have its repercussions. Women, mostly the vocal, articulate and inquiring middle-class women who had so eagerly accepted in the 1920s and 30s that hospital birth was the safest way, began by the 1960s and 70s to query the quality of the birth experience supplied by the hospitals, and to query their safety statistics. Jane Lewis, in her book *The Politics of Motherhood*, sums up the changes in attitude thus:

> It would be impossible to decide whether the decrease in infant mortality could or should be weighed against a subtle strengthening of the ideology of motherhood, or better medical care in childbirth against the loss of control by women over its management. But it is important to be aware that all this has happened and that neither

changes in medical practice nor in social policy, both of which were important in determining the shape of maternal and child welfare services, can be assumed to have been benevolent.[66]

The questioning of the direction in which the birth process has gone, in Britain and much of Europe and certainly in America, has prompted many 'new' philosophies of birth. In the context of history, many of these may be seen to be not so much new as a change in emphasis made possible by the simple fact of radical and wide-ranging developments in medical technology and skills.

MEDICAL CHANGE

In attempting to assess the profession's response to public criticism it would be easy to forget the fact that obstetricians in general, and British obstetricians in particular, have made greater efforts to monitor the quality of their work than most other specialities within medical practice.[1]

In the twentieth century, work done in various areas of general medical research had enormous importance for the field of obstetrics. Directly relating to women and reproduction was the growth of understanding of fertility and the reproductive processes, particularly menstruation. For centuries ignorance and superstition, modesty and cultural taboos had placed menstruation outside the field of constructive research. In the twentieth century, at last, these barriers were put aside, opening the way to a greater understanding.

Chemotherapy, a new science, was made possible by the discovery of the sulphonamides; and the groundwork was laid for the discovery and development of penicillin and other antibiotics. This work, in turn, was only possible because of the preparatory work done on bacterial causes of disease by scientists like Pasteur, Koch and Domagk. Advances in haematology — prevention of clotting and the establishment of blood groups — made blood transfusion a realistic possibility and both minimised the risk of death from haemorrhage and made surgery safer. This, in conjunction with the development of the science of anaesthesia, allowed major advances in gynaecological and obstetric surgery.

Many other fields were opened up to the progressive researcher: radiology, clinical pathology, endocrinology, microscopy, ultrasound and the assessment of the wellbeing of the fetus *in utero*. Understanding of anatomy and physiology led to a completely new branch of obstetric care — the treatment of infertility. Virology opened the understanding of the way in which chromosomes work, and genetics developed as a science.

Much of the work done has made medical knowledge more complete. It has also made it more complex and sophisticated, requiring a greater degree of specialisation among doctors, and in some areas raising questions which are not merely medical but ethical and moral as well. This is perhaps particularly true in the area of reproduction and fertility, where efforts are made not just to preserve or sustain life, but also to engineer or create it.

Old Problems Solved

Sepsis

Infection was always one of the most persistent problems of childbirth. By the end of the nineteenth century the presence of microbes was accepted, but neither their genesis nor the mechanism by which they passed from person to person was clearly understood. Nor, finally, did there exist any treatment for sepsis.

The foundation of the work of discovery had been laid down by Paul Ehrlich, whose search for a selective germ killer, a 'magic bullet', culminated in 1910 in the discovery of Salvarsan 606, which cured the virulent venereal disease, syphilis. The chemical treatment of bacterial diseases, however, was only successful up to a point. Ehrlich's pioneering work was taken up and developed by a scientist called Gerhard Domagk, who had gained the appointment of director at the giant German chemical organisation, I G Farbenindustrie.

Domagk's goal was to achieve with plant-like micro-organisms what Ehrlich's arsenic compounds had achieved with animal germs. Some of Ehrlich's early research had employed the selective dyeing of tissues, and one of his early 'magic bullets' was a dye called trypan red. Domagk took chemicals in the sulphonamide group, and found that they had the property of dyeing particularly colourfast — that is, they bonded exceptionally well with the cells in fabrics. Would they bond as well with cell tissue? In 1932 two chemists working at the plant manufactured the chemical from which the red dye *Prontosil rubrum* was obtained. Domagk began to test the effectiveness of the dye on thousands of mice, injecting them first with large doses of streptococci, then countering the injection with a dose of *Prontosil.* The dye worked and the mice, which should have been killed by the streptococci, survived. Eventually the chemical compound in the dye which was responsible for killing the germs was isolated.

The sulphonamides provided a vital stepping stone in the fight against bacteria. The struggle against the virulent haemolytic streptococci was extended in a grand manner by the discovery of penicillin by Sir Alexander Fleming, and by its development as a drug by Howard Florey and Ernest Chain.

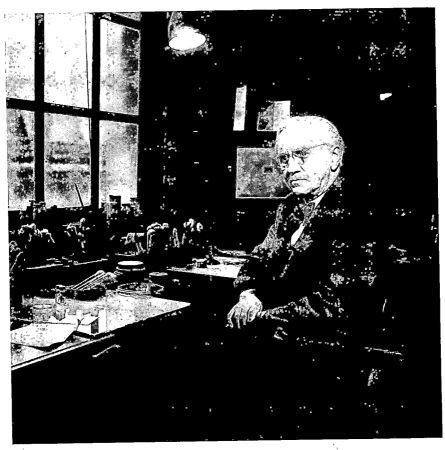

Sir Alexander Fleming, who discovered the penicillin bacteria.

To Fleming goes the credit of perceiving the possibilities of penicillin as an antibacterial agent; but he found that it was unstable, unreliable and lost its effectiveness quickly, and he abandoned attempts to develop it as a drug. Ten years later the Second World War broke out in Europe; and the need for antibiotics effective against the terrible wound infections that were the result of the conflict became pressing. In Oxford Howard Florey and his assistant Ernest Chain began to look again at Fleming's records; and they set themselves to consider how the culture could be developed to act *within* the body rather than merely on the surface, as Fleming had considered it.

The most important immediate result of their work was the discovery that penicillin was harmless to the white blood corpuscles and did not affect their powers of resistance. In addition, they discovered that the drug was passed quickly through the system and evacuated through the urine, so that large doses were required for effectiveness. Clinical trials proceeded with all speed, and Florey published his results in 1941.[2]

Now that the knowledge was available, it would have seemed a simple step to put the drug into production; but Britain, hard-pressed by her war efforts, simply did not have the technological resources for such production, and it was not until an invitation was forthcoming from the United States to the English scientists to continue their work in that country that production on a large scale became possible. Thereafter, penicillin began to be used extensively. After the war it was found to be effective in the treatment of puerperal fever. The discovery and development of penicillin represented a major step forward in medical history. (Tragically, the establishment in Britain was against the taking out of any patents on the drug; in consequence, Britain has lost a fortune in revenue which might well have been channelled into other areas of medical research.)

While work was proceeding in research into the development of antibiotics, parallel work was being undertaken on the nature of streptococci themselves. After the identification of the various strains of bacteria, it became possible to trace the source of infection. Studies in the

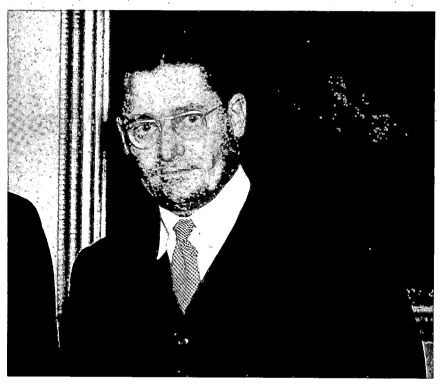

Sir Howard Florey, who was responsible for developing penicillin as an antibiotic.

1930s[3] showed that many cases of puerperal fever had resulted in the transference of bacteria from the nose or throat of the doctor or attendant. Further studies showed that haemolytic streptococci were capable of surviving in dust for several weeks.

It became apparent that between 30 and 40 per cent of women harboured anaerobic streptococci (bacteria which flourished without oxygen) in the upper vagina during late pregnancy and early labour. The likelihood was that organisms found in the genital tract originated in the intestine; injury to the birth canal if operative obstetrics were required made the likelihood of infection greater. Thus, although the discovery of effective antibiotics greatly reduced death from puerperal fever, the gradual general improvement in obstetric skill — notably in Caesarean section — after 1930 made infection by this route more likely.

Once the strains of bacteria had been identified, and particularly after the discovery of the sulphonamides and of penicillin, treatment of the fever was possible. Prophylactic measures were also possible, and new antiseptic routines were introduced.

Haemorrhage

In childbirth women always ran the risk of haemorrhage. Great and rapid blood loss would lead almost inevitably to a state of surgical shock and thence to death. The introduction of ergometrine to speed the delivery of the placenta and cause the blood vessels to contract helped in this respect; but work on blood transfusions was hindered by two major problems: first that the blood clotted; second that a reaction was often noted when certain blood was donated.

The problem of clotting was finally solved in 1914 by Albert Hustin in Brussels by adding sodium citrate to hinder coagulation. The problem of compatability was complex. It had been shown in 1874 that the blood of one species of animal can 'attack' and break down the cells of another, thus causing death; but it was not until 1901 that the Viennese Karl Landsteiner — who was later also responsible for research into Rhesus incompatibility — announced his discovery of agglutins in the blood (the clumping of blood corpuscles) and classified human blood into four groups. He demonstrated that the blood serum in one group of blood might cause the agglutination of the red corpuscles in another group.

By 1915 it was possible for the surgeon to give the correct blood to his patient, and in a manner that did not cause clotting. Yet blood transfusions as a widespread method of treatment did not become possible until the 1930s when blood banks were set up. In 1921 a voluntary donor system set up by the Red Cross in London was developed into the London Blood Transfusion Service, and other such organisations began to spring up in larger cities around Britain. But once again it took the advent of war to galvanise a more sophisticated system of blood donation and storage into existence. These systems set up through the exigencies of war laid down the pattern for future development, and a national blood donation scheme was organised.

Pain Relief

Anaesthesia, which became available to some women in the late nineteenth century, represented painless childbirth, and women had suffered in birth for long enough. So it was pressure from women, in tandem with the efforts of obstetricians like Sir James Young Simpson, that encouraged further research into analgesia and finally made the use of pain relief commonplace in labour.

It was recognised by the end of the nineteenth century that choloroform, because of some dangerous side effects, was not the ideal anaesthetic, and the search for a safe painkiller went on. Around the turn of the century, work was begun in Germany on the effects of a mixture of drugs, scopolamine and morphine, which were administered by injection. Twilight Sleep, as this cocktail was dubbed, became popular in America and Britain in the 1920s and 30s, largely as a result of pressure from certain groups of women. The early moves were made in America, where feminist and suffragette groups pushed unremittingly for pain relief. For example, a Boston homoeopathic doctor, Eliza Taylor Ransome, began the New England Twilight Sleep Association in 1914 to try to force hospitals to adopt this method of pain relief. Brochures published by the Association advertised that it 'abolished the need for forceps, shortened the first stage of labour, and helped the mother produce milk; it was the best method for women with heart trouble and with "nerves"'.[4] By the 1920s, hospitals in Boston had adopted this method of pain relief, and in the next twenty years Twilight Sleep had become almost universal.

There were, in fact, considerable drawbacks to Twilight Sleep. Attempts to introduce a standard dose in order to minimise the calls on attendance did not prove satisfactory. The required dose was different for every woman, and there was no such thing as a standard dose. In many women it was noticed that considerable time elapsed between the administration of the first dose and the patient's passing into Twilight Sleep, and drugs other than morphine were introduced to try to combat this — nembutal, sodium amytal and pernocton. Pernocton induced sleep, scopolomine was given immediately after it, and when the patient awoke she passed into the 'Twilight' state.

Twilight Sleep fell into disuse, as chloroform had before it, when other more satisfactory drugs were tested and eventually came on the market.

sleep; and analgesics relieve pain, while not necessarily causing drowsiness. Most drugs will cross the placenta and affect the baby in a similar way to the mother. The timing of administration as well as the dosage given are therefore important and must be carefully judged.

The development of pain relief in obstetrics has had many effects other than the obvious one of reducing the amount of pain suffered by women in labour. It has been instrumental in placing ever greater control of the birth process in the hands of doctors and has taken birth into the hospitals where facilities are available. It has tended to increase the incidence of intervention in labour and delivery — while at the same time opening the way to the improvement of surgical techniques. Lastly, and ironically, many of these effects have driven women to reject the very relief they had sought so assiduously only a few decades previously.

Changes in medical practice

As the move to the hospitals increased, doctors became ever more aware of the kind of damage that a complicated delivery could cause; and the attention of the medical profession turned increasingly towards the notion of prevention. To the medical mind, it seemed logical that the often severe gynaecological problems which doctors were required to treat surgically after delivery should be avoided in the first place. So began a new era of medical intervention in the birth process — not, this time, from 'granny' midwives eager for their beds, nor from families desperate to shorten the long labour pains of their nearest and dearest, but from doctors and obstetricians, and mostly for the most humanitarian of reasons.

Routine intervention in the birth process was advocated by Joseph B DeLee of Chicago. In an article published in 1920 entitled 'The Prophylactic Use of Forceps', he recommended the routine use of forceps and episiotomy. DeLee suggested that the 'patient' should be sedated; that ether should be given when the fetus entered the birth canal; that the perineum should be cut for several inches between the vagina and anus to prevent spontaneous rupture during birth, and that forceps should be applied to the infant's head through the perineum. The fetal heart should be monitored by stethoscope, and ergot or a similar agent would be used to hasten the delivery of the placenta, which would then be extracted with a 'shoehorn maneuver'. The perineal cut would then be stitched.[5] According to DeLee, prophylactic obstetrics prevented many kinds of damage which were greatly feared by mothers — damage either to themselves or to the fetus: prolapsed uteri, vesico-vaginal fistula or sagging perineums, babies with epilepsy, idiocy or cerebral palsy. His treatise was widely influential in America, and by the 1930s prophylactic obstetrics had there become the norm.

In Britain, too, the trend in the 1920s was towards increasing medical intervention in birth, though the doctrine of prophylactic obstetrics never had quite the influence it did in the States. The necessity of strict aseptic procedures, though, was strongly emphasised, and attention was focused more and more on abnormal rather than normal labour. Labour was, women were told, 'a major surgical procedure'.[6] Certain routines became the norm; for example, shaving and disinfection of the vulva was regarded purely as a possible pre-operative procedure in 1906, but by 1930 shaving was common practice and aroused, it seems, no great objections. The Medical Women's Federation Maternal and Child Welfare Committee recommended 'a tightening up of the technique of the preparation of the patient for labour, eg the giving of an enema, shaving the patient, etc.'[7]

The position of delivery changed too. In Britain it had been usual for a woman delivering to lie on her left side, the position that Victorian attitudes had pronounced the most modest. By the 1920s, leading obstetricians were recommending that women lie on their backs with their feet in rests — a position which made surgery easier, but which was much more likely to cause perineal tearing.

DeLee's recommendations for the 'prophylactic use of forceps' reflected a growing interest in the health and condition of the fetus: a new interest made possible by the increasing ability to prevent maternal mortality. The new science was dubbed 'perinatology' — the care of the infant in late pregnancy and the first week after birth. Perinatology brought with it a whole new set of medical interventions; the increase of induction of labour, monitoring of the fetal heartbeat and the use of episiotomy numbered among them.

Induction

Artificial induction of labour was hardly a new feature of birth intervention; for centuries it had been employed either for motives of self-interest, particularly by 'granny' midwives anxious to get off home, or for medical reasons, such as preventing the mother from having to carry an over-large fetus. In America in the first decades of this century, it was not uncommon for labour to be hastened so that the delivery of a smaller baby would make the labour easier for the mother. There was no consideration of the possible effect on the child:

> Nothing pleased me more in my obstetrical work than to have the baby born a week or two ahead of time . . . Consequently it is not unusual for me to try to 'shake the apple off the tree' ahead of time by castor oil or quinine, or by starting labour with a rubber bag . . .[8]

By the 1940s and 50s, however, it had become not uncommon for 'fetal indication' to be taken into account when assessing the need for obstetric intervention. That is, doctors began to intervene in the birth process for the sake of the child, even if there were no signs of distress in the mother. By 1941, the American Gynaecological Society had come down strongly in favour of intervention to assist the fetus:

> More babies and mothers will be injured by undue prolongation of labours that fail to progress than by timely operative interference.[9]

Research carried out in the 1950s and 60s gave doctors more and more information about the well-being of the fetus in the womb. Tests were evolved that determined the role of the placenta and examined its efficiency in specific cases. Once techniques had been developed to listen to the fetus's heartbeat, such checks became a standard component of antenatal care. Fetal heart monitoring during labour emerged in the 1960s, using either electrodes fixed to the scalp of the fetus, or an ultrasound transducer placed on the mother's abdomen to pick up the fetal heartbeat. Now that the obstetrician was able to check on the continuing efficiency of the placenta, whether the lungs were sufficiently mature for a reasonable chance of survival, and whether the fetal heart was sound and strong, intervention 'for the sake of the fetus' became not only possible but in many views desirable.

The 'active management of labour' became very much a feature of modern obstetrics following the synthesis of oxytocin and the development of the prostaglandins. An American called Emanuel Friedman presented in the 1950s a series of articles on 'graphostatistical analysis' — computations of the average length of time taken in labour by women of various obstetrical histories. From these averages, with their upper and lower limits which formed to Friedman 'a norm', he concluded that

> It is clear that cases where the phase-durations fall outside of these [statistical] limits are probably abnormal in some way.[10]

A 'partogram' was devised — a chart which plots the average rate of dilatation of the cervix and descent of the fetus. If labour did not follow the chart to the satisfaction of the obstetrician, a drip was set up to speed up or slow down the process. This process is not as simple as it might sound. One of the disadvantages of using an oxytocin drip to speed up labour is that it tends to increase the strength and frequency of contractions, making pain relief more or less essential. If pethidine or a similar drug is administered to counter the pain, this will in turn slow down the contractions. In order to speed them up again, more oxytocin is given; this in turn causes greater pain . . . and so on.

This particular type of intervention reached its height in Britain in the 1960s and early 70s, when induction became not merely a means of protecting mother or fetus, but quite simply a means of achieving the convenient administration and smooth running of the hospital. In 1974, 38.9 per cent of births in England and Wales were being induced.[11] Yet 1974 had seen widespread debate about the wisdom of a policy of wholesale induction, and an article in the *Lancet* in that year concluded that 'until unequivocal evidence is available, the public is right to question medical practices of doubtful validity that are based on convenience.'[12] And two years later Danae Brook was writing:

> Having been introduced for very good reason, induction for social convenience is now being encouraged by some gynaecologists, and a number of hospitals have tried to bring a policy of 'nine to five deliveries' because they fear that shortage of night staff might endanger the night-born babies. However, according to the English medical paper the *Lancet*, there is some evidence that babies born during the day might be more 'vulnerable to the kind of distress that requires oxygen administration'.[13]

Research has now shown that there is a high incidence of fetal distress connected with large doses of oxytocin. An American study found that a slowing down of the fetal heart rate was more common in induced labours, 'due to a greater intensity of contractions and counter pressure on the fetal head caused by greater resistance of the birth canal'.[14] There is no predetermined 'correct' dose of oxytocin.

By the early 1980s, the fashion for induction for convenience had almost passed, certainly in Britain. There is no sure way of judging that the time is right for induction, and 'there will inevitably be a proportion of cases in which an error in dating of gestation results in a premature child who may die or suffer irreparable damage in the neonatal period'.[15] In America in 1967 the induction rate was roughly 9 per cent of all births; in Britain it rose from 27 per cent in 1970 to 33 per cent in 1972, and as high as 40 or 50 per cent in the mid 1970s.

While induction rates have since fallen considerably, the principle of 'active management of labour' is still very much pursued in the National Maternity Hospital in Dublin. Here every labour is actively controlled, while the mother is guaranteed a labour of no more than twelve hours and the constant presence of a midwife. The principles of management as laid down (by Kieran O'Driscoll, the obstetrician behind the practice) are rigidly applied. Obstetrical intervention is relatively low.

Episiotomy

Another obstetric intervention which was not new but which began to be undertaken 'for fetal interest' was episiotomy, the cutting of the perineum.

Episiotomy was first described by Fielding Ould in 1742:

> There must be an incision towards the anus with a crooked pair of
> probe-sizars; introducing one blade between the head and the vagina
> . . . and the business is done at one pinch, by which the whole body
> will easily come forth.[16]

The intention was to avoid the kind of massive tearing of the perineum
between vagina and anus that would be a source of great pain and
embarrassment to the mother.

In some countries, episiotomy was quite common well before the
1930s, although Britain was notably conservative about the operation. In
America, where the delivering woman lay on her back with her feet in
stirrups, tearing was particularly likely and episiotomies therefore
became common quite early.

After the 1930s, the operation was considered to expedite speedy
delivery, and its incidence grew rapidly:

> The fetus is to be protected from the effects of a prolonged second
> stage, particularly from certain injuries which may result when the
> head acts as a 'dilator' [of the perineum].[17]

Williams, a standard textbook on obstetrics, refers to episiotomy for the
first time in 1950: it 'spares the baby's head the necessity of serving as a
battering ram'.[18]

By the time of the Second World War episiotomies were routinely
administered to all first mothers in the United States, and the likelihood
of subsequent deliveries requiring the operation was high. By the 1970s
episiotomies had become common practice in most western hospitals. By
this time, midwives were allowed to infiltrate the perineum with local
anaesthetic in order to perform episiotomy; prior to this, many
episiotomies were carried out completely without an anaesthetic.

In the late 1970s and early 80s, the trend was being reversed, and many
women today are rebelling against the routine performance of
episiotomy. There is no substantial evidence for the advantages of the
operation in most circumstances — although, plainly, episiotomy is
preferable to a third-degree perineal laceration; by contrast, it is clear
that women who have not had episiotomies experience less pain at the
end of the first week after delivery, have fewer breastfeeding problems
and experience less discomfort from intercourse.[19] Reams of advice have
been forthcoming regarding preparation for a birth without episiotomy
— by antenatal massage of the perineum, exercises and healthy diet; and
in labour by the use of hot compresses, hot baths and massage.

Caesarean section

During the present century, another form of medical intervention has

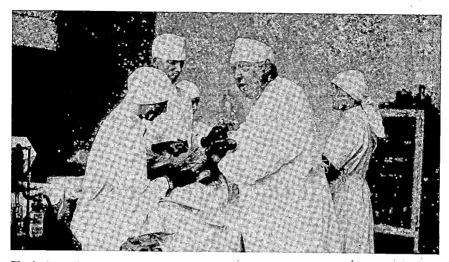

Techniques in surgery saw many changes in the early years of this century. Here Sam Cameron from Glasgow is seen operating using rubber gloves – face masks are not in use.

become both possible and increasingly common — delivery by Caesarean section. The refinement of the techniques of Caesarean delivery in the early years of the century made for many mothers and their babies quite simply the difference between life and death. Caesarean section by the end of the 1920s had become a reasonably safe operation — an acceptable alternative, in fact, to the high forceps operation. In Britain in 1929, even at a time when death of the mother from Caesarean section was as low as four per cent, there remained a reluctance to perform a section in the case of placenta praevia (when the placenta obstructs the birth canal):

> 'The fetal mortality in these cases was necessarily very high,' said one doctor in defence. 'It is probable that some of these infants might have been saved by Caesarean section, but the important point is that, from the mother's point of view, operation was unnecessary.'[20]

The dangers of the operation were, of course, compounded by the absence of proper blood transfusion methods.

In Glasgow in the 1920s, 'there was an average of two maternal deaths every week, and we were so preoccupied with the problem of keeping the mother alive that the high fetal mortality rate was never discussed.'[21] In that city between 1925 and 1929 there were 226 deliveries following craniotomy; 11 per cent of the mothers died.

Gradually the percentage of Caesarean deliveries undertaken has risen. Many factors have been associated with this rise; in the highly litigious American society, the threat of malpractice suits has been the foremost

175

reason. The general clinical indications for the operation have also widened considerably over the last decade: where once section was performed in cases of disproportion, pre-eclampsia and placenta praevia, indications are now taken to include poor obstetric history, placental insuffering and fetal distress. Where once breech presentations were normally delivered vaginally, as many as 40 per cent were delivered by Caesarean section in 1982. And the early dictum 'once a Caesar always a Caesar' has not yet been entirely dropped by the medical profession; the rise in the primary Caesarean section rates means that there is inevitably a still greater rise in subsequent, repeat rates.

In recent years there has been, alongside the growing Caesarean section rates, a greater awareness of the emotional, as well as the physical effects of the mother and the mother-child relationship. The importance of 'bonding' has been examined, and the difficulties of bonding after a Caesarean birth, particularly where a general anaesthetic had been used. Also, the statistics concerning vaginal birth after Caesarean (VBAC) have been seriously questioned,[22] and now more and more women are safely giving birth to their second and subsequent children after an earlier section.

Caesarean section, like so many 'modern' obstetric developments, has undoubtedly on many occasions saved lives and made possible a safe delivery where before mother and baby would have died. The whole paraphernalia of modern medicine combined to give women the chance of a 'safe' pregnancy and delivery.

Maternal mortality dropped dramatically, and the new attention to the well-being of the fetus made a woman entering pregnancy expect that at the end of it she would be well and healthy and have a well and healthy baby.

All that after centuries of pain, fear and infection, and a high risk of death or damage! And yet . . . to many women it seemed that something was wrong.

THE TIDE TURNS

> A woman was powerless in the experience of birth and unable to find meaning in it, for her participation in it and even her consciousness of it were minimal. She was isolated during birth from family and friends, and even from other women having the same experience. . . . She played a social role of passive dependence and obedience.[1]

From the mid 1960s, it became apparent that many women were beginning to question the experiences they were having in hospital, to evaluate them, and to ask themselves: Is this what birth is all about?

But the questioning had been triggered much earlier, and one of the first people to question the meaning and quality of the experience of birth was not a woman but a male doctor: Grantly Dick Read. Dick Read worked for many years among mothers in slum areas in London in the 1940s, and his work there convinced him that there was more to motherhood than the aseptic, sterile, anaesthetised conveyor-belt system that the hospitals were offering. His feelings became crystallised finally on a visit to Whitechapel in the early hours of the morning:

> In due course the baby was born. There was no fuss or noise. Everything seemed to have been carried out according to an ordered plan. There was only one dissension: I tried to persuade my patient to let me put the mask over her face and give her some chloroform when the head appeared and the dilation of the passages was obvious. She, however, resented the suggestion, and firmly but kindly refused this help . . . she shyly turned to me and said: 'It didn't hurt. It wasn't meant to, was it doctor?'[2]

The incident had a telling and lasting effect on Dick Read. For years he struggled to understand the apparent paradox: that motherhood, the beautiful culmination of love and marriage, could not be meant to hurt — but that it undoubtedly and commonly did.

The theory he came up with became known as the fear-tension-pain syndrome:

> Fear and anticipation have given rise to natural protective tensions in the body, and such tensions are not of the mind only, for the mechanism of protective action by the body includes muscle tension. Unfortunately the natural tension produced by fear influences those muscles which close the womb and prevent the child from being driven out during childbirth. Therefore, fear inhibits; that is to say, gives rise to resistance at the outlet of the womb, when in the normal state those muscles should be relaxed and free from tension . . . The implementation of my theory is demonstrated in the methods by which fear may be overcome, tension may be eliminated and replaced by physical and mental relaxation.[3]

Dick Read's teachings about 'natural childbirth' were a revelation to millions. To a generation of women who had been brought up in relative ignorance about the process of birth, and who were given to understand either directly or by direct inference that childbirth was massively painful, his teachings of self-knowledge came fresh out of a cloudy sky. To women who had been so sedated that they remembered the birth of their child — if they remembered it at all — through a haze of analgesia, his descriptions of the mystical experience of birth itself seemed the promise of a new era:

> I have been told that no woman should see her baby until it has been bathed and dressed. My patients, however, are the first to grasp the

> small fingers and touch gingerly the soft skin of the infant's cheek.
> They are the first to marvel at their own performance . . . It is a
> moment when, in the full consciousness of their achievement, they
> experience a moment of intense emotional joy.[4]

In Britain, the beginnings of questioning about the need for medical
intervention and the routine administration of analgesia had already
become noticeable by the late 1930s. One matron in a large maternity
hospital said

> For a long time after I became matron I failed to understand why so
> many women asked to be looked after by the nurses and not by the
> medical men who attend the hospital . . . The reply I had was
> astonishing. 'Because the doctors all make us have chloroform
> whether we want it or not, and the nurses don't!'[5]

According to Dick Read, the suggestion that pain existed was enough in
itself to bring on pain. It was not part of his teaching to insist that women
should undergo birth without having the chance of pain relief; merely
that a woman, properly educated in 'natural childbirth', would have no
fear and would therefore be less likely to require pain relief:

> To tolerate suffering when it can be relieved is no less brutal than to
> insist on suffering when it is not present . . . The administration of
> anaesthetics and analgesics should have definite indication in
> obstetrics as it has in every branch of medicine or surgery. Pain is the
> only justification . . .[6]

In Britain, Dick Read's ideas caught on, and 'natural' childbirth by
preparation before labour and encouragement and support throughout
labour became a real possibility for many women. In 1956 the National
Childbirth Trust was formed to bring Dick Read's ideas to a larger
number of women; and although many consumer groups have since
sprung up, the NCT has been the most broadly influential lay movement
in Britain. In the United States, where Dick Read's ideas were well
received by American women, they were not as successful in practical
terms. Dick Read's methods depended very largely on constant contact
and support throughout labour; in American hospitals this seemed to be
impossible:

> The majority of women who attempted to follow Read's advice did
> so under hostile conditions. They shared labour rooms with women
> who were 'scoped' [scoplomine/morphine] and their screams,
> combined with the repeated offerings of pain relief medication by
> the hospital staff, reinforced the very fear of birth that Read had set
> out to remove.[7]

At the same time, many women interpreted Dick Read's ideas in terms
of 'success' if labour proceeded without pain relief, and 'failure' if

medication was given. Opponents of the 'new' birth insisted that these pressures on women to 'perform' led to the marked increase in post-natal depression in the 1950s. Feminist writers like Betty Friedan, on the other hand, interpreted such depression as a consequence of the realisation by women of the emptiness of their lives as homemakers, particularly in the period following the birth when they discovered that motherhood did not provide all the satisfaction and fulfilment that had been promised.[8]

If Dick Read's ideas were less successful in the States than in Britain, they did nevertheless correspond with a period of questioning about the 'birth experience' in that country. Many women felt that there should be more to giving birth than merely being dragged down into the dark valley of unconsciousness, surfacing finally to be presented with an infant with whom they felt no ties, no bond. It was clear that if women were to regain any control over their birth experience within the American system, a new approach was needed.

It came, unexpectedly, via Russia. There, following World War Two, doctors began to develop ancient folk practices, counteracting pain signals by the concentration of the mind on extraneous sensations — 'psychoprophylaxis'. In 1951 this was adopted in Russia as the 'official' method of pain relief. Two French doctors, Pierre Vellay and Ferdinand Lamaze, studied the method in Russia and developed it further, adding to the counter signals a rapid, shallow breathing system that became known as the 'Lamaze method'.

Painless Childbirth, Lamaze's book, appeared in 1956. An American woman, Marjorie Karmel, who lived in Paris at the time, wrote of her experience of the Lamaze method in another book, *Thank You, Dr Lamaze*; and it was her book that effectively introduced the Lamaze method into the United States.[9] Karmel, together with a physiotherapist, Elizabeth Bing, and a doctor, Benjamin Segal, founded a new pressure group, ASPO — the American Society for Psychoprophylaxis in Obstetrics. The group was geared to American institutions and their methods of birth management — and it left control firmly in the hands of the doctor.

The Lamaze method nevertheless represented a new departure in the approach to childbirth. Preparing for the birth experience, practising breathing and the controlling of contractions provided a new, *active* role for women. For the first time since the beginning of the takeover of birth by the medical profession, birth was not simply something that happened to you; it was something that you actively participated in. The 'scientific' basis of the method appealed to women, and the method became one of the cornerstones of the new feminist movement. Women were beginning to regain power in the place of birth.

Around the mid 1960s, another birth philosophy began to make its appearance, again in France. Dr Frederique Leboyer was 'Chef du

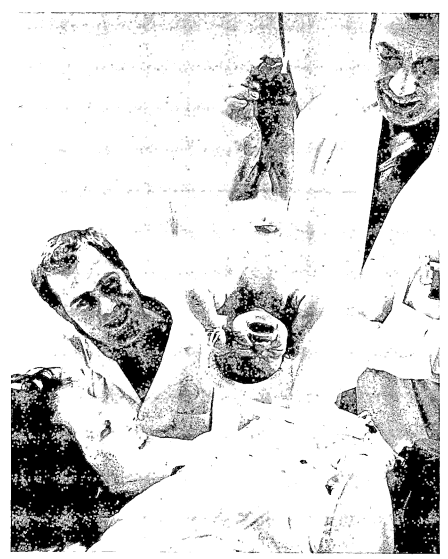

'A small creature has just been born. The father and mother gaze at it with rapture. Even the young assistant looks pleased.'

Clinique' in the Paris Faculty of Medicine; and he turned his attention away from the labouring mother and focused it instead on the newborn infant.

'Pictures of newborn babies are horrible; they look like tortured prisoners,' argued Leboyer.[10] He painted a vivid picture of the birth room:

A small creature has just been born. The father and mother gaze at it with rapture. Even the young assistant looks pleased. One dazzling smile lights up their faces. They radiate happiness. All of them, that is, except the child. The child? Oh, dear God, it can't be true! The mask of agony, of horror . . . can birth hold so much suffering, so much pain? While the parents look on in ecstasy, oblivious.[11]

Leboyer's plea for a consideration of the welfare of the baby was a far cry from the purely medical concern that had evolved during the 1930s and 40s. This was a plea for a different kind of birth, and *Birth Without Violence* was a love-poem to the newborn child. Birth was to be gentle, lights dimmed, voices soft. The baby was to be placed on its mother's stomach and gently massaged. It was to be immersed in body-warm water, a simulation of the fluids it had just left. Leyboyer, however, was not quite the first to write in this vein. Maria Montessori, around 1930, was writing in much the same tones about the newborn baby:

He arrives in the adult world with delicate eyes which have never seen daylight and ears which have never known noise. His body, hitherto unbruised, is now exposed to rough contact with the soulless hands of an adult who disregards that delicacy which should be respected . . .[12]

Others, too, had suggested that more thought should be given to the emerging infant; yet it was Leboyer's book that made the greatest impact — perhaps because women, now more aware of their own bodies and more in control of the birth experience, were ready to turn their attention to the well-being of their babies.

While many women were delighted by Leboyer's views, his profoundly 'poetic' way of looking at birth nevertheless disturbed many others. Obstetricians with their modern 'medicalised' approach to birth found it impossible to accept what seemed to them a dangerous fantasy:

I believe that we have enough real problems to solve during labour without indulging in ritualistic daydreams leading to activities of more than questionable usefulness . . . I find the whole business quite superfluous since . . . it absolutely directs the attention of the obstetrician toward tasks which may well distract them from the essentials of their skill.[13]

Nor have male doctors been the only critics of Leboyer: feminists have viewed his approach as 'contemptuous' of women:

. . . he does not trust us to respond in a tender loving way to our own newborn. It is left for a male, medical professional to create an artificial rite of passage for the natural one we could create if we were not denied the opportunity.[14]

Others have seen Leboyer's own participation in the birth event as a modern example of the 'couvade' ritual of primitive tribes, where the husband imitates his wife's pregnancy and birth symptoms:

> The symbolic re-emergence from the amniotic fluid and the
> rebirthing by the father's hands is the male improvement over the
> female's birthing.[15]

One early result of Leboyer's work — and one considered by many
women to be unfortunate — was that some obstetricians began to adopt
the superficial, cosmetic aspects of a 'Leboyer birth' while retaining
complete medical control of the entire process:

> The band-aid approach he [Leboyer] takes leaves itself open to being
> co-opted out of any meaning. It is possible right here in Boston to
> have a 'Leboyer birth' (quiet, dimly lit room, massage, bath to relax
> and recreate the womb experience) along with an epidural fetal
> monitor, and perhaps your 'drug of choice'.[16]

One gynaecologist who was profoundly influenced by Leboyer was
another Frenchman, Michel Odent. Odent, concerned to move as far
away as possible from birth as a medical event, recognised the futility of
the cosmetic approach:

> ... birth without violence is not a method, a technical modification
> which can be rapidly and easily assimilated by means of some
> indeterminate reform. It is a development in concepts, a
> revolution.[17]

With this in mind, Odent developed a special unit at his hospital in
Pitheviers in France, building up a team of like-minded staff to support

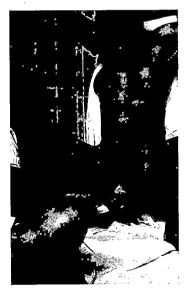

A woman gives birth in the 'salle sauvage' at Pitheviers.

his work. He began, in his own words, to 'demedicalise' birth, creating a birthing environment free of all the paraphernalia of modern medicine, and encouraging the mother to adopt standing or squatting positions for delivery:

> In our 'salle sauvage', our birthing room at Pitheviers, the dorsal position seems out of place . . . [it] is harmful because it compresses important veins, goes against gravity, doesn't allow for pelvic expansion, the perineum doesn't stretch as it should, and retained amniotic fluid can be a source of infection.[18]

One novel innovation was the introduction of bathing pools, available for the use of the labouring mother:

> We never plan in advance to use water or not to use it. Sometimes, though, labour may be long and painful . . . We have found water can help a mother to release her inhibitions and let her cognitive brain go . . . We don't know what water actually does to the body. It may loosen gelatinous matter in the tendons. Sometimes just looking at the water or hearing running water is enough to release a mother's tension, and the baby is soon born.[19]

Odent considers forceps obsolete, and uses analgesia rarely:

> When you use a drug during labour you destroy a complex hormonal equilibrium in the mother's body. It is virtually impossible to recreate such complex interaction using drugs on the mother.[20]

Recourse to Caesarean section, even for such widely accepted indications as breech birth or previous section, is rare.

Odent's methods may still be extreme within the medical profession, but they have led to a move, however tentative, towards a new compromise: birth within the hospital environment, with all the latest technology to hand, but kept at bay as much as possible. The trend is represented, for example, by the introduction of 'birthing rooms' at some hospitals — often at the suggestion of midwives — where natural childbirth is encouraged.

A more determined 'demedicalisation' of the birth process had begun in the United States before the advent of Leboyer and Odent in France. It had begun on two fronts: by feminists, concerned that women should regain control over their bodies, their fertility and their ability to give birth without male-dominated aid; and by women whose views were based on tradition — the dream of a woman, snug in the bosom of her family, giving birth in a natural way to another member of that family.

Furthering the interests of such groups was a new breed of birth attendant, the lay midwife. One of these was Raven Lang, who was among the first to document an approach to home birth which grew from the 'pro-feminist, pro-natural lifestyles, anti-war and anti-establishment climate of the counter culture of North California in the late sixties'.[21]

The home birth movement was seen by some women as the only possible way of escaping the hospital-dominated, male-dominated American way of birth. In Tennessee a group of people, concerned to find a new communal, vegetarian, quasi-religious way of life, set up a self-supporting commune called 'The Farm'. To reinforce their lifestyle, they sought to recapture lost skills of midwifery. Long study and much practice resulted in a book, *Spiritual Midwifery*, which has had a widespread and profound influence on the growth of the American home-birth movement.

In Britain, birth at home declined continuously through the 1960s and 70s, largely as a result of pressure from the authorities for hospital delivery and the gradual running down of domiciliary services. In 1979 Sheila Kitzinger — who was possibly the first woman to have an extensive influence on modern birth movements — presented her study, *Birth at Home*. Her book was a soundly researched look at the place of birth. She stressed the importance of good health, a proper home environment and good obstetric history as prerequisites for home birth, and was far from uncritical of the hospital recipe for birth:

> It is sometimes taken for granted that any hospital is safer than any home. This is entirely a false assumption. There are excellent hospitals where a high-risk baby has the greatest chance of being born safely, but there are others which are badly staffed, poorly equipped, haphazardly run, in which the progress of labour is inadequately observed and the woman left for long periods during which no-one is aware of what is happening to her.[22]

Kitzinger was critical of the standardisation of procedures in large hospitals, and of

> . . . iatrogenic, or doctor-produced illness, which in turn calls for more intervention. The more iatrogenic malfunction that is produced, the more necessary do doctors seem.[23]

Whether hospitalisation of birth has achieved greatly improved perinatal mortality statistics, as the doctors claim, or merely implemented 'iatrogenic malfunction', as Kitzinger insists, it is certainly true that home birth in the Britain of the 1980s is the exception rather than the rule, with only about one per cent of all births taking place in the home. Official reports have ignored the question of women's preferences in this matter, subordinating them to what the respective committees viewed as the best policy:

> . . . the understandable preferences of mothers in regard to the place of delivery may not be compatible with the requirements of maximum lowering of perinatal and neonatal mortality.[24]

So by the 1980s, control by the medical profession of the birth process, from antenatal care through to delivery, had become such that women's wishes were seen as irrelevant, medical judgement supreme. Reluctance by the authorities to permit birth in the home has led to the setting up of schemes such as the 'domino' scheme ('domiciliary midwife in and out'). The compromise effected in this scheme is that the birth takes place in the hospital, but all antenatal and postnatal care is undertaken by the local midwife, who takes the mother into hospital when delivery is imminent, and takes her home again shortly after birth.

Opposition by obstetricians to birth in the home is, by and large, implacable; yet there are countries in the western world which run a system where home births represent a high proportion of all births. One such country is Holland, where home births account for around half the total number of births. From the early years of this century, there have in the Netherlands been special training programmes for maternity-aid nurses, whose role has been to help the mother in the home during the lying-in period. She works alongside the midwife, who undertakes total care of the birth process; and the midwife works in tandem with the local doctor. Thus for all normal, healthy women, birth took place — and still does — in the home; while for those considered in some way 'at risk', the hospital provides further care.

In Holland, as in other countries, the prerequisites for home birth are considered to be the absence of 'risks', and every year the indications for hospital delivery grow more numerous, antenatal checks more stringent. In addition, the Dutch system works well both because highly trained domiciliary midwives have never been phased out and because there is easy access in most parts of the country to local hospitals in case of emergency. Despite pressure from outside influences, Dutch women apparently still prefer birth at home:

> The advantages of home confinement are that in her own home the expectant mother is not considered a patient, but a woman, fulfilling a natural and highly personal task. She is the real centre around which everything (and everybody) revolves. The midwife or doctor and the maternity aid nurse are all her guests, there to assist her. This setting reinforces her self-respect and self-confidence. The modern hospital very often functions in the opposite way . . .[25]

Whatever the reason, Dutch perinatal mortality statistics prove that the system is not only workable but also produces acceptable results. Compare, for example, the perinatal mortality rate for births outside hospital in 1975 (4.1 per thousand) with the figures for the same year in Oklahoma (52.6 per thousand) or California (42.3 per thousand).

Studies made of home births in the United States and in Britain,[26] however, have suggested that 'the current technological trend in childbirth does not have all the solutions and that other options such as home delivery need to be examined.'[27]

The 'consumer revolt' against the 'medical revolution' has been represented not just by the spontaneous growth of home-birth movements, nor merely by the proliferation of literature on the subject. Consumer organisations and pressure groups began to make their appearance. In Britain the emergence of the National Childbirth Trust promoted a new approach to labour, birth and maternity care generally. The organisation was originally designed for the education of women, teaching them to understand what was happening to their bodies, and instructing them on how to relax and deal with pain.

AIMS, the Association for the Improvement of Maternity Services, was founded in 1960 — originally under the name Society for the Prevention of Cruelty to Pregnant Women — to improve maternity services generally. Its early enthusiasm for improved technology in childbirth was replaced before too long 'by an awareness of the price that often had to be paid by mothers and babies for the use of the new techniques'.[28] The stand of the organisation was expressed by one writer in 1978:

> What a pity it is that childbirth, that most creative and joyous of events, should have become in the last few years a battle-ground, to be fought over by opposing factions whose only common characteristic, seemingly, and yet the one that divides them most deeply, is a sincere desire to do what is right.[29]

AIMS makes a plea for the right of maternal choice — to have a baby free from interference 'unless she wants it or there are clear indications that it is needed'.[30]

Such organisations served to raise popular consciousness about the evolving status of birth; and in 1974 public debate increased following a highly critical report by the Oxford Consumer Group on birth practices. The debate centred then on the induction of labour, and was heightened and sustained by press coverage.[31] In Durham, Margaret Whyte, conscious of the difficulties that were encountered by women wishing to have their babies at home, set up her Society to Support Home Confinements. The Maternity Alliance, describing itself as a non-partisan forum, was founded in 1980 to provide better services for mothers and babies in Britain; the Active Birth Movement was founded in 1982, another alliance of 'consumers and care-providers'. The Association of Radical Midwives was established by a group of midwives working within the National Health Service who were worried about the diminishing role of the midwife, and who believed that 'only through extended and improved midwifery can we achieve any real progress'.[32]

The proliferation of childbirth literature and the rapid growth of consumer movements in the field demonstrate quite clearly that, while the 'medical revolution' of the twentieth century has been a phenomenon without parallel, it will take very many years for its impact to be assimilated and for the new technology to assume its rightful place in the area of childbirth.

THE GROWTH OF ANTENATAL CARE

> The first step ... in the direction of successful treatment of the unborn infant must be successful treatment of the pregnant mother.[1]

Little in the way of real medical attention to antenatal care existed in the nineteenth century but, by the turn of the century, particularly in America, there were noticeable efforts being made in this area. In Boston in 1901 the Instructive Nursing Association began to make antenatal visits to outpatients in Boston's Lying-In Hospital. By 1912 the Association was making a minimum of three antenatal visits to outpatients. In 1909 an experimental intensive prenatal care programme was started in Boston by Mrs Lowell Putnam of the Infant Social Department of the Women's Municipal League of Boston; women registered to be delivered at the Boston Lying-In Hospital were visited every ten days by a nurse, instructed in the hygiene of pregnancy and given emotional comfort and reassurance. In May 1911 the pregnancy clinic at Boston was opened to outpatients.

The attention to prenatal care was triggered by the discovery that pre-eclampsia could be controlled by rest, diet and drug treatment, and that adequate prenatal care could help to pinpoint its onset. Once in care, the monitoring of urine and blood pressure could minimise the development of eclampsia. Other tests such as the Wasserman test, which diagnosed maternal syphilis, could be performed prenatally, and any necessary treatment carried out. (More recent studies indicate that antenatal care may not be such an effective means of diagnosing pre-eclampsia as the early antenatal care champions thought.)

In Britain at the beginning of this century, antenatal care was more or less non-existent, although health visiting had begun as early as the 1860s. Dr John William Ballantyne of Edinburgh, a specialist in fetal pathology, was the pioneer of antenatal care in Britain. His work on fetal pathology had set him wondering if anything could be done to prevent abnormalities by better care before delivery. As Ballantyne saw it, 'the first step ... in the direction of successful treatment of the unborn infant must be successful treatment of the pregnant mother . . . [but] the profession does not understand the physiological changes of pregnancy.'[1]

Ballantyne began to believe in 'pro-maternity' care: and following the presentation of his paper 'A Plea for a Pro-Maternity Hospital' in 1901,[2] the first antenatal bed — called the 'Hamilton Bed' in tribute to that early

Edinburgh pioneer of medical midwifery, Alexander Hamilton — was set up in Edinburgh's Royal Infirmary. Despite this move, however, few hospitals would admit a mother before the onset of labour, and the paucity of pre-maternity beds in Britain made the treatment of complications of pregnancy very difficult.

. Ballantyne envisaged that pre-maternity beds would give the opportunity for study and research into the abnormalities of pregnancy and the newborn which hitherto had been impossible. Enthusiastic about the work being carried out in Boston, Ballantyne instituted a scheme in Edinburgh whereby a trained nurse would visit pregnant women at home, give advice, test urine and look for any danger signals, and would then report any such signals to the doctor back at the hospital. The system worked for a short while, then was superseded by a hospital antenatal clinic system in 1915.

· The first outpatient clinic — so legend has it — also opened in Edinburgh. A local doctor, Haig Ferguson, was in charge of women in a hostel for unmarried pregnant women in Edinburgh. All the women, who were admitted into his care in the sixth or seventh month, seemed to have fine, healthy children. Ferguson was convinced of the need for medical supervision for improving maternal and infant health and well-being. He made his Presidential Address to the Edinburgh Obstetrical Society in 1912, emphasising the importance of 'intra-uterine puericulture'.[3] In his view, 'rest before confinement, good food, healthy surroundings and avoidance of excitement, seem to give the mother greater vitality, more perfect nutrition, full-term labours, and good recoveries.[4]

By the middle of 1915, a small antenatal clinic had opened:

> The premises in which these clinics are held consist of one room, divided into two by means of a wooden partition, and lavatory accommodation in the basement of the hospital. There is a separate entrance from a side street, which is on a level with the basement. The patients wait in the outer half of the room, and are seen by a doctor in the inner half. The consulting room is rather noisy and not very well lighted, having one window of translucent glass. Artificial lighting is by means of gas; the floor is covered with linoleum; a coal-grate and a sink are fitted in the doctor's room.[5]

Not a very impressive beginning, perhaps, but a beginning nevertheless.

The first official steps to provide antenatal care had been taken in 1914 when the Local Government Board issued a circular containing details of an antenatal scheme to be carried out at infant welfare centres. These guidelines were not implemented by many authorities until after the 1918 Maternity and Child Welfare Act. The scheme catalysed the distrust that lay at this time between the GPs, midwives and local authorities. Midwives feared that they might lose their patients to the hospitals if

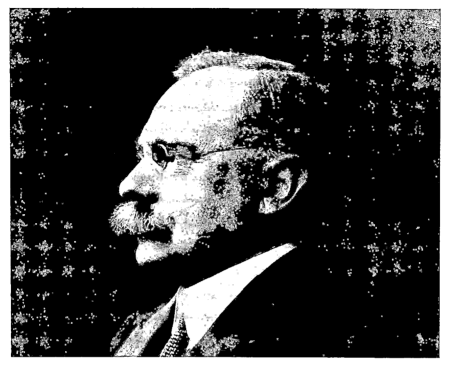

J W Ballantyne, the Edinburgh pathologist who introduced the concept of antenatal care.

they referred them to hospital clinics for antenatal checks. In 1918 *Nursing Notes* advised midwives that they were under no obligation to co-operate with the local authority clinics should they not wish to do so. These problems were not finally sorted out until after 1936, when a salaried service for midwives was introduced by the local authorities.

On the other hand, the British Medical Association felt that the GP should be in charge of antenatal care, and that clinics might threaten his fee. A statement issued in 1929 read, 'The Association is firmly of the opinion that the usual routine work done at these centres can be done quite as well at the consulting room of the doctor or in the home of his patient.'[6]

Opposition by GPs to the clinics was not supported by women's groups, who were strongly in favour of the continuance of the clinics and of the extension of their work. In 1931 it was found that the cost of expanding the work of the clinics was less than the cost of implementing a GP antenatal service, so the clinics remained. Yet financial stringency made the expansion of the services — or even attempts to maintain them at their existing level — extremely difficult. The number of clinics throughout the country, however, increased from 120 in 1918 to 1,931 in

1944. The proportion of pregnant women attending these clinics rose to 76 per cent in 1944, and almost 99 per cent two years later.

The service provided by the clinics varied widely from area to area; some clinics advised five or more visits, others endorsed the recommended minimum of two visits only. Some authorities used the clinics more or less as an extension of the education services, offering mothers classes on mothercraft. Others would ascertain the expected date of delivery and position of the fetus, but not bother to do blood or urine tests. Little actual medical treatment was provided, only attempts to relieve minor pregnancy ailments.

A number of hospitals ran their own antenatal clinics. At Glasgow's Royal Maternity Hospital Mary Thomson, student midwife, took her turn at the clinic:

> I took the large basket and went around collecting specimens. And from the depths of shopping bags, handbags and pockets, there emerged an astonishing array of vials, pill bottles, beer and whisky bottles, pickle and sauce bottles, lemonade and squash bottles, each carrying its own story and very often providing a deep mystery to the tester when their original contents had been insufficiently washed out.[7]

At this hospital the clinic was used as a means of tutoring students, the doctor

> holding short tutorials in each cubicle by examining the patient first and then asking one of his students to examine her and tell what he had found . . .[8]

Another of the duties of the hospital clinic was to ascertain whether venereal disease was present, so that it could be treated as quickly as possible:

> Great tact had to be used in handling patients, for in those days it was almost a criminal offence to suggest that anyone had venereal disease . . . I once asked Sister what I would tell the patients who asked me about the VD on their cards, and she said ... they wouldn't understand anyway, for most of them thought Venereal was something for eating.[9]

Generally speaking, women were slow to take advantage of antenatal care. Middle class women, in particular, felt that in some way such care was associated with illegitimate births (oddly, the emphasis has now swung in completely the opposite direction, and now the likelihood is that working-class mothers or unmarried mothers are the slowest to take up antenatal care). Some authorities felt that pregnancy should be 'notifiable' as were infectious diseases. (Notification of *births* became compulsory in 1907.) Women's groups felt strongly that this was too much of an intrusion into private life, and preferred that women should be educated into using antenatal facilities.

Education was, perhaps, really needed, for many women were still shy about pregnancy, and particularly embarrassed about the thought of internal examinations by doctors. There were relatively few women doctors available for this kind of work. Moreover, many women were deterred by the impersonal treatment meted out by antenatal clinics, and by the long hours of waiting in queues. Indeed, the routines of antenatal care even by the 1930s were still haphazard. The average number of visits by a pregnant mother might vary from one or two to three or six. Some clinics might ascertain fundus, lie and presentation, listen to the fetal heart, take blood pressure and a urine sample. Pelvic measurements might be made, but some records show that they seldom were.[10] Blood tests were seldom given although by 1949, blood tests appeared to be more widespread.

The nature of antenatal care has changed very considerably as the technology available to the doctor has grown. Central to the improvement of the detection of fetal genetic or growth problems have been the development of cell culture from amniotic fluid (where a sample of fluid is drawn off from the sac surrounding the fetus) and the invention of ultrasound.

By the early 1950s, very little had been accomplished in one major area

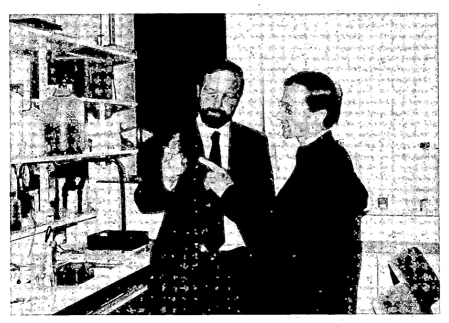

David Brock (left) and Roger Sutcliffe perceived a link between a high level of alphafetaprotein and spina bifida.

191

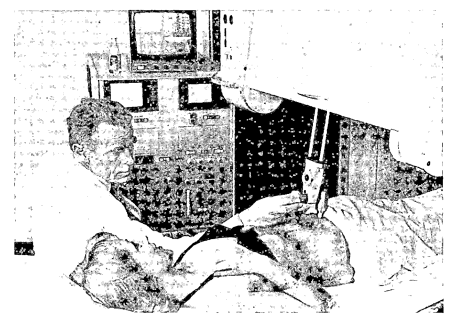

Professor Ian Donald from Glasgow developed ultrasound scanning.

of research — prenatal diagnosis. Almost nothing could be told about the condition of the unborn child. A doctor or midwife could feel a pregnant woman's abdomen with the hands, and describe the position and size of the fetus. But its sex, health or possible growth defects or abnormalities remained a secret to be shrouded until birth. In the 1870s scientists working in the field of obstetrics had begun to examine the amniotic fluid in the hope of finding information about the genetic make-up of the baby. The operations they performed were on women who had died in pregnancy. It was not until 1919 that the first amniocentesis was performed on a living mother, and not until the 1960s that a method was discovered of cultivating the cells found in the fluid — cells which had been shed by the fetus. When this had been done, the chromosomes they contained could be examined under a microscope, and certain genetic information gathered. As new techniques are developed, more and more information can be gleaned in this way — for example, the detection of spina bifida through the presence of a high level of alphafetaprotein (afp), a link established by Edinburgh researchers David Brock and Roger Sutcliffe in the 1960s.

At this time, however, the task of performing an amniocentesis was necessarily a hazardous one — 'pray and plunge' as it was described. The location of the placenta became possible through the development of another major innovation, ultrasound scanning. Ultrasound took over from X-radiography (which had proved so harmful) as a means of visualising the fetus in the womb. Picking up on submarine detection work during the First World War, a Scots doctor called Ian Donald began to use the technique of targeting ultrasonic frequencies (frequencies greater than 20,000 per second and beyond the range of human hearing) at the fetus *in utero*. Sound vibrations travel at different speeds in different substances; where they cross the interface between two substances, some of the energy is reflected, some transmitted. Echoes from the interface can be recorded in visual form on a cathode ray tube or on a television screen. The technique took some time to develop, but it is now in widespread use in many countries throughout the world. Although there have been many doubts raised about the possible dangers of ultrasound scanning during pregnancy, there has never been a long-term study of its possible risks. Nevertheless, it is thought that, unlike X-rays, low energy ultrasound is non-ionising, and does not harm the tissue.

In the hospitals, routines changed to accommodate the ever increasing number of mothers using the new techniques of care. In America as early as the 1940s, hospitals in the large cities were structured for maximum efficiency. To ensure that everything ran smoothly, staff were encouraged to control patients passing through the system, to precondition them to the idea of trust and obedience, so that when the time came for labour and birth they would not prove 'troublesome'.

Weight control was used as a means of social conditioning. Medically speaking, it was thought that keeping excess weight gain in check contributed to the prevention of pre-eclampsia. In fact, excess weight

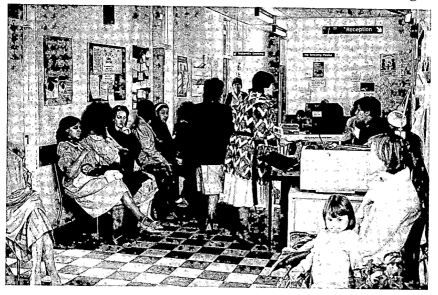

An antenatal clinic in 1983. Scenes such as these are a familiar part of the birth process in Britain.

gain is a sign of pre-eclampsia, not a precondition of it. However, patients were 'judged' by staff as 'good' if they contained weight gain to around twenty pounds, and 'disobedient' or 'troublesome' and 'morally inadequate' if the doctor's orders were 'disobeyed' and weight rose rapidly or too much. Notes would be taken to the effect that the patient was 'troublesome'. Antenatal routines preconditioned the patient to accept other hospital routines that were to follow as 'what were best for the baby'. Patients were often kept isolated from each other and therefore more dependent on hospital staff.

Antenatal care, once accepted, became absorbed into the generally increasing 'clinicalisation' of the childbirth process. Throughout the early years of the century, emphasis was placed by successive governments counselled by committees heavily influenced by consultant obstetricians on the need to treat the birth process more and more 'scientifically'. Even when women's groups pointed to the harsh economic and social conditions that lay behind maternal and perinatal mortality, the response was to examine only the clinical and medical reasons for death.

As recently as 1978 Roland Moyle, Minister of State for Health, said 'It may be that social conditions are the predominating influence on this problem [of perinatal mortality], but I am determined that health care will make its maximum contribution.'[11] The Short Committee, set up to study perinatal and maternal mortality, reported in 1980 that the number of handicapped babies could be reduced by about five thousand, and between three thousand and five thousand deaths prevented 'if modern knowledge and care are universally applied.'[12]

The emphasis would appear still to be on clinical care, even though research has indicated that social and environmental factors have at least as great an influence on obstetric performance as does obstetric care.

Comparisons between mortality in Britain and in neighbouring countries — Holland, Denmark and Sweden — were established in 1932 when a delegation of experts was sent to investigate their superior statistics. They recognised that the problems which earlier industrialisation had brought to Britain — notably overcrowding and smoke pollution — did not exist to the same extent in the other three countries. Diet also appeared to be better than in Britain; and in those countries, the midwife still enjoyed a large measure of involvement in the care of pregnancy and birth, whereas in Britain doctors had to a large degree taken over.

The clear evidence that social and environmental factors greatly affect obstetric performance was paralleled by comparisons of regional statistics within Britain itself; and the importance of *long-term* improvement in diet and health has been emphasised by recent work showing that average height is greater in prosperous areas — and obstetric performance is improved in taller women:

> While advances in medical care will probably continue to reduce the perinatal mortality rate, it is unlikely that rates similar to those in Sweden can be achieved until a generation of women has been reared in an environment comparable to that in Sweden where social class differences in stature have disappeared.[13]

In a time of high unemployment, there are today many areas in which diet is poor. A single woman living on social security, for example, could not hope to purchase the food recommended for a pregnant woman. And in areas of high unemployment, perinatal mortality figures are also high. In addition, women living in stressful conditions may try to deal with pressure by turning to the comforts of alcohol or cigarettes, both of which they are told endanger the health and well-being of the fetus. The knowledge that they are doing something harmful to their baby leads in turn to further stress, as does pressure at antenatal clinics to turn away from such comforts:

> . . . the advice they gave on smoking confirmed their fears, and transformed pregnancy from the carefree and enjoyable time they had anticipated into one of anxiety and apprehension.[14]

Care, it seems, should be judiciously meted out.

Certainly modern techniques of prediction and visualisation have made it possible for much greater care and attention to be paid to the health and well-being of the fetus — although a knowledge and an understanding of problems at an early stage in pregnancy can pose a new set of problems for parents and doctors, and a new set of worries. Nor, despite ever-improving mechanical aids, can human fallibility be eliminated. In one study

> An analysis of the rate at which asymptomatic problems are diagnosed, missed and overdiagnosed . . . indicated that detection of some problems is incomplete and that overdiagnosis is common. The productivity of routine antenatal care in respect of prediction and detection of obstetric problems is extremely low . . .[15]

Overdiagnosis could lead to 'overinvestigation and unecessary admission, induction or operative delivery'[16] and tests can be a great worry to parents waiting to hear their outcome. One doctor wrote

> I know of women who have found their level [of AFP] was high and the period of uncertainty that followed so harrowing that they have vowed never to be screened again.'[17]

Other studies have shown widespread effects of stress on women and their partners waiting for results:

> 'If they are inside you and you're worrying terrible it must affect them somehow.'
> 'My husband's greatest worry was that the baby was perfectly normal but I would miscarry because I was so worried . . .[18]

In addition to these problems, it was plain that the women who were most likely to attend antenatal clinics were middle-class women in good health; single women or women from lower social classes who were potentially more at risk tended to start their antenatal care later and make fewer return visits:

> ... dissatisfaction may be one of the reasons for the high defaulting rate in some groups. It is likely that visits which are unproductive, arranged with poor continuity and hurried will be unsatisfactory both for the pregnant woman and the attending staff.[19]

The question of dissatisfaction has rested on a number of issues; excessive workloads at many clinics have caused long waiting times followed by brief consultations; there has been general lack of continuity of care, the mother rarely seeing the same doctor or midwife on successive visits. Women questioned in a recent survey[20] found the travel to a central hospital expensive and inconvenient, the waiting times unnecessarily long, the staff brusque and unsympathetic — often merely because they were too busy to give individual attention. Mothers with other small children found making arrangements for their care during hospital visits a problem, and there were no facilities at the hospitals to care for or amuse toddlers.

On the other hand many women — especially those who had been identified as being 'at risk' — often found the hospital staff both helpful and pleasant:

> 'Sometimes there was a long wait but every care was taken, when you actually got to see the doctor, to explain what was happening to you and your baby.'
> '... the gynaecologist is the most king and sympathetic person i have ever met during my pregnancies.'
> 'It was reassuring going to the hospital clinic; everyone made me feel relaxed and important . . . as soon as you went in to one of the doctors, you immediately got the impression that you were the only person that he was going to see that day.'[21]

Many women, though, felt that:

> '... the attitude of many doctors insults the intelligence of mothers. We are entitled to know what is happening to our unborn child; tests should be explained.[22]

Many, too, felt that the emphasis of the hospital was too clinical:

> ... the mothers were just carriers for his healthy babies and not important in themselves. I think he would be happier if he could grow babies in his laboratories!'[23]

The burden of work placed on hospital antenatal clinics means that many women find them inadequate; doctors have insufficient time to answer their questions or sense their emotional needs. The awareness that emotional, as well as physical, needs are important in caring for the pregnant mother was summed up in a book published as long ago as 1970:

> As obstetrics has developed from an art to a more scientific speciality in the last three decades, there is a suspicion that some may overlook the fact that childbirth is a normal physiological function . . . the lowest perinatal mortality rates cannot be achieved without technical efficiency, but the quality of a service should be considered in humanitarian terms as well as those of efficiency.[24]

All of this seems to call into question the relevance of antenatal care as it exists today: but clearly antenatal care does have benefits — and considerable ones in some cases. Every 'at risk' mother whose problem has been identified and dealt with as a result of antenatal screening will testify to this. There are many lessons to be learned from such criticisms of the system as listed above, and some are being implemented through official channels, albeit slowly.

In antenatal care, as in the rest of the field of obstetrics care and birthing, the centuries-old battle for control between midwives and the medical profession is still very much current. The sharing of antenatal care — between hospital consultant and his obstetric team, the GP and his team of community nursing staff — was recommended in various reports from the 1960s onwards. Recognition of a need for wider co-operation between the maternity care services, however, did not necessarily bring with it such shared care. A maternity co-operation card for women having shared care was introduced in some places as early as the 1960s, but it has taken decades to achieve anything like widespread usage.

Today, certainly, a large number of people may be involved in antenatal care: the mother, the consultant obstetrician, the general practitioner, the midwife, the health visitor, the liaison health visitor, the paediatrician, the family planning service, the dietician, the dentist, the social worker, the physiotheraptist and the community medicine specialist. Shared care, particularly shared between the general practitioner and the hospital, with the emphasis in normal cases on attendance at GP clinics, is far from unusual. In some areas, special attention has been given to the development of particular kinds of shared antenatal care. One such scheme is located in Sighthill in Edinburgh, an area where there was for a long time a poor record of attendance at antenatal clinics and a concomitant unacceptable perinatal mortality record. Here, the midwife and the GP share between them all antenatal care of most of the pregnant women in the district, each having his or her own list. Once a month a consultant obstetrician from a nearby teaching hospital joins the team and reviews the 'at risk' women. Few mothers are likely to have to attend the hospital antenatal clinic, and community involvement in the scheme is encouraged: care is taken into the home if there is difficulty or reluctance to attend the clinic. The improvement of mortality figures since the implementation of the scheme is noticeable.

New patterns of antenatal care have, in fact, become evident in many areas, often making greater use of the midwife and community clinics. In 1982 the Royal College of Obstetricians and Gynaecologists Working Party on Antenatal and Intrapartum Care also suggested that the number of antenatal visits should be reduced, to five for low-risk women. Only by such a reduction could the demand for improvements in the general running of antenatal clinics be carried out, claimed the report.

The aims of antenatal care were spelt out in a document published in 1929 as follows:

1 to predict 'difficult labour' from examination in pregnancy;
2 to detect and treat toxaemia;
3 to diagnose/treat/prevent infection (e.g. dental, cervical);
4 to diagnose and treat VD;
5 to ensure that 'the closest co-operation' between the clinic and all persons in charge of pregnancy care;
6 to recognise 'the educational effect of a well-organised clinic'.[25]

Current aims of antenatal care may have changed little, but there are many questions still to be asked about the general effectiveness of the present system of care, its cost, and the tendency to put screening programmes above general improvements in the standard of living as a means of improving perinatal mortality.

FERTILITY AND CHOICE

The promotion of childbearing cannot be separated from its prevention.

> Anne Oakley, *The Captured Womb*, p253.

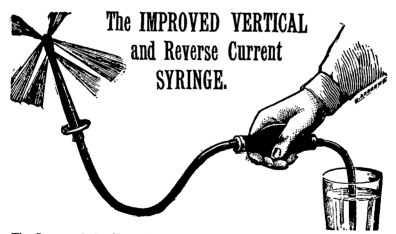

The **IMPROVED VERTICAL and Reverse Current SYRINGE.**

The Improved Appliance is a powerful Enema of Higginson's pattern, fitted with a new Vertical and Reverse Current Vaginal Tube. producing a continual current treble the power of the ordinary tubes used for this purpose, thoroughly cleansing the parts it is applied to. It is to be used with injection of sufficient power to destroy the life properties of the spermatic fluid without injury to the person, and if the instructions are followed it can be used with success and safety.

Complete in Box, with particulars for Injection, aud directions for use,

Post free, 3/6 and 4/6 each.

THE EVOLUTION OF BIRTH CONTROL

> The just and proper use of these methods must be described as ethically positive. Everything is moral which makes for the happiness and well being of society: everything immoral which prejudices or endangers it.[1]

> I trust you will agree with me in the hope that . . . the medical profession ... must never identify itself in this matter ... if this evil is to continue, it shall never exist as a sidewing of the healing art.[2]

Some means of controlling the population rate has been practised in most societies as far back as history records. In communities where the natural death rate was high, there was obviously a need for continual replacement of the population and thus for a high birth rate. Sometimes, however, special conditions — famine, for example, or other circumstances of great hardship — would force a community to try to limit its population in some way in order to make the best possible use of its resources.

Not all methods of population control related to interference with the reproductive cycle before conception. Abortion, by a great number of methods, was always one option; and in many communities, notably India and China, infanticide was widely practised, and to a certain extent still is. It would often be the female children who were the victims. Sometimes children with severe handicaps were killed at birth, or babies were sacrificed for ritualistic or religious reasons.

Other communities practised male castration. It has been known for thousands of years that the removal of the testes of the male at puberty will diminish or totally remove his sex drive and impair the development of secondary sexual characteristics — his voice would not break, and there would be little growth of body hair.

In ancient China, it was believed among the upper classes that if a man slept with many women without ejaculating, his seed would be much stronger when he attempted to fertilise his wife. This ancient form of *coitus reservatus* involved stern self-discipline, and aids such as pretending the woman was grossly ugly, or 'gnashing the teeth a thousand times' were employed.

In other societies, attempts were made to divert semen by other means. Infibulation, whereby the foreskin was pulled down over the penis and held in place with a metal ring, was certainly employed in Roman times. One group of Australian aboriginals practised male sterilisation by making an incision under the penis so that the semen was carried out through it rather then entering the woman's vagina. This was undertaken around puberty, and practised on the laziest, weakest or most wicked of the tribe, ensuring the survival of the fittest and most worthy.

More common were attempts to provide a barrier around the entrance to the vagina in the form of a pessary of some kind. An Egyptian manuscript dated around 1850 BC tells of a recipe involving a paste made from crocodile dung. A later paper records a concoction made from honey and the hearts of the acacia plant. This recipe might have had some efficacy: honey has a clogging effect much like oil and would have inhibited the mobility of the sperm, and acacia tips ferment to form lactic acid — a sound basis for spermicidal jellies.

In ancient Greece, operative procedures were sometimes resorted to. The historian Strabo records that women of the court often had their ovaries removed so that they might preserve their slim figures. Infanticide and abortion were widely practised in ancient Greece and Rome, too, for large families were frowned upon in better families. Aristotle recommended the use of frankincense mixed with olive oil placed inside the vagina; the Roman physician Soranus published a list of plants believed to be effective as contraceptives, and a list of materials for use as pessaries. He warned against the use of irritant materials and scorned the notion of charms, incantations or potions. Other suggestions were less well founded: he recommended that after intercourse a woman should squat down and sneeze to attempt to expel the semen from the vagina. He also suggested that if a woman held her breath at the moment of male orgasm, the semen would not enter the cervix. The notion that if a woman does not experience orgasm, but instead tightens her vaginal muscles, she will not conceive, persists even today.

Soranus was no expert on contraception, but many of his ideas at least had some foundation. By the Middle Ages they had been lost, and many ideas apparently prevalent at that time now seem merely ludicrous. Pessaries made from elephant dung, animal ear wax or cabbage, or the fumigating of the vagina with the smoking hoof of a mule, all sound as unpleasant as they are ineffective.

Many methods of 'contraception' were based on pure superstition. The woman might wear an ornament, such as the foot of a weasel, the finger of a dead fetus or the anus of a hare, hung around the neck. Magic potions might be drunk, containing such strange ingredients as iron rust, potter's clay or the kidney of a mule. Herbs naturally played a large part in the recipes — thyme, lavender, parsley, asparagus, willow leaves, and numerous others. Chants and incantations were also used, or the new bride would sit on her fingers, hoping to be free from pregnancy for a number of years that corresponded with the number of fingers she chose to sit on.

It has to be remembered that several factors affected women's fertility in the past that do not affect western women today; girls usually began to menstruate later, and their general life expectancy was considerably shorter. Many women would never live to experience the menopause.

After puberty, there was every likelihood that a woman would spend a considerable part of her life either in pregnancy or breast feeding. Breast feeding — at least when milk is given freely on demand — provides a fairly effective means of suppressing ovulation. Carl Djerassi, one of the scientists who worked on the development of the pill, asserts that, '. . . even now, when considered on a global scale, *more births are prevented by breast feeding than by any other method of contraception*.'[3] But until the middle of the nineteenth century, little was really understood about the reproductive process, and attempts at contraception were always something of a hit or miss.

Coitus interruptus, withdrawal before orgasm, was undoubtedly used from time immemorial, and is still widely used today. The Church, however, did not approve; taking as its doctrine the teaching of St Paul, it gave the procreation of children as the only justification for sex, and quoted Genesis in condemnation of withdrawal:

> Onan . . . spilled the semen on the ground, lest he should give offspring to his brother. And what he did was displeasing in the sight of the Lord, and he slew him also.[4]

By the sixteenth century, however, texts indicate that it was possible for at least some women to enjoy sex with some freedom, as long as their

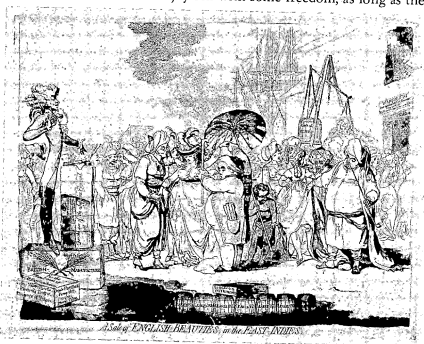

A Sale of ENGLISH BEAUTIES in the EAST INDIES

A bale of condoms in this 1789 cartoon by Gillray shows that long before vulcanisation of rubber, London did a roaring trade in condoms.

men withdrew in time: 'Disport yourself and give me pleasure,' wrote one fun-loving lady, 'but take care not to sprinkle me inside, not with a single drop, or it will be a matter of life and death.'[5]

Coitus interruptus remained a major means of avoiding conception until the emergence of a rapidly thriving industry in the marketing of contraceptive devices in the second half of the nineteenth century, as Germine Greer has pointed out:

> One of the effects of British imperialism was a plentiful supply of cheap rubber, which became expensive rubber when it was formed into sheaths and cervical caps. The flood of literature instructing gullible buyers in contraceptive methods which began in the 1870s was largely subsidised by the manufacturers of contraceptive hardware, and we cannot be surprised to find that it had little to say for a method which used no hardware at all.[6]

Coitus interruptus has nevertheless remained popular as a method of avoiding conception — it is, after all, free, instantly available, and accessible to all.

Another method of contraception which did not rely on manufactured apparatus was the so-called 'safe period'. That the cyclical nature of female fertility should long have been grasped is not surprising, although many thought the fertile time was during bleeding. It was not until the 1930s that the details of the ovulation/menstruation cycle were fully understood. The 'safe period' is still a wildly unreliable method of avoiding conception, even if fairly precise calculations are made.

Exotic pessaries were one of the earliest of artificial devices designed to prevent conception. Soranus in the second century described a number of such pessaries, some of which might have had some degree of efficacy had he not recommended withdrawal after two or three hours, before intercourse took place. Indeed, over the centuries, it was the question of *when* to put in a pessary that seems to have vexed physicians. Nineteenth-century literature, however, shows a resurgence of interest in these devices. Allbutt's *The Wife's Handbook* advertised an own-brand of quinine pessaries at two shillings per dozen:

> There is nothing but quinine and cocoa-nut butter in these pessaries, consequently nothing to irritate either the woman's vagina or the male organ.[7]

The pessaries could be made over the kitchen range with the aid of half a pound of cocoa butter, 5 dr borax, 1 dr salicylic acid and 1 dr of quinine bisulphate, the whole to be cooked slowly and the sticky fudge that resulted to be cut into suitable-sized pieces ready for use.

A big advance in contraception came with the introduction of the condom. A sheath, worn as a protection for the penis, was probably in use long before the first reliable records of the device in 1564. At that time it was largely worn as a means of avoiding syphilis or other venereal disease. It would be made from linen, and later from a dried bladder or a section of intestine from some animal. It was not considered for contraceptive use until around the eighteenth century.

No one really knows the origin of the word 'condom'. A *Tatler* of 1709 claimed that:

> A Gentleman of this House (Wills Coffee House) . . . observ'd by the Surgeons with much envy; for he has invented an Engine for the Prevention of Harms by Love Adventures, and has, by great Care and Application, made it an immodesty to name his name.[8]

The notion of a 'Mr Condom' inventing the device and giving his name to it has a certain appeal, but seems unlikely. More plausibly, it may be derived from the Latin *condere*, to protect. The English nickname 'French letters' may derive from the fact that many of these devices were washed up on the south coast beaches — 'letters' from France.

The manufacturers of condoms grew in steady proportion to their rise in popularity. Styles changed too, and the linen device which so inhibited sensitivity was abandoned in favour of a fine animal membrane, often tied with ribbon. In 1740 a man called Thomas Streetser, writing as 'Roger Pheuquewell Esq.' wrote his bawdy 'A New Description of Merryland' (the vagina). Visitors were asked to wear 'proper Cloathing' to protect them from the 'dangerous heat of the Climate'. This was to be made of an 'extraordinary fine thin substance, and contrived so as to be all of one Piece and without a Seam, only about the Bottom it is generally bound round with a scarlet ribbon for Ornament.'[9]

The making of these eighteenth-century condoms was an elaborate process involving long soaking in alkaline solutions and washing, scenting and polishing as well as tieing on decorative ribbons. Wetting the device before use made for a better fit, and James Boswell often describes in his memoirs how he 'engaged in armour',[10] performed 'safely sheathed' and once how in St James's Park he 'dipped his machine in the Canal and performed most manfully'.[11]

Britain soon became an international centre for the sale and distribution of condoms. In the 1840s a shilling booklet, *On the Use of Night Caps* publicised their use. It recommended putting 'over the gentleman's gentleman a very fine nightcap . . . Let it be tried *on*, and the experiment would not be found complete without its being tried *in*.'[12] The vulcanisation of rubber in the mid-nineteenth century brought an increase in the popularity of the condom, until by the 1930s in America it accounted for almost one-third of all types of contraception used.

The sponge is perhaps the oldest type of barrier contraceptive. Known to have been used in the time of Christ, the sponge was mentioned in the Talmud, but fell into disuse. The next known reference was in 1600, when a French prostitute was discovered to have in her possession not only a probe, ointments and a syringe but also a sponge. By 1786 in France, at least, the sponge was commonplace as a means of contraception:

> You wet this sponge in water mixed with a few drops of brandy; you insert it exactly over the mouth of the womb, so as to block it; and even if the pervasive semen goes through the pores of the sponge, the extraneous liquid, mingling with it, destroys its power and essence.[13]

Around 1823, handbills distributed in Britain show that the sponge was popular here too; and Marie Stopes, proponent of contraception in the 1920s and 30s, was distributing the sponge at her clinics — albeit somewhat patronisingly:

> Women who have been examined and found, for some reason or another, to be physically, environmentally or mentally not quite up to the standard of the occlusive cap, are taught to use the sponge... though a few may object to its clumsiness, none can find it harmful.[14]

Recent work has made a modern sponge available on the general market.

The cap may have been pioneered in the early eighteenth century by Casanova, who described the cutting in half of a lemon, the extraction of the juice, and the wearing of the half-segment in the vagina. Lemon juice would certainly have been an effective spermicide, but the entire operation sounds most uncomfortable. In 1838, a German named Wilde designed a cervical cap, made from a wax mould of the patient's cervix, then fashioned precisely in ivory or gold, silver or latex. Interestingly, a new cap, called the Contra cap, has recently been developed, fitted in the time-honoured way by taking an impression of the cervix. A one-way valve allows the escape of the menstrual flow and mucous secretions.

The cervical cap was in use for many years, though it never achieved widespread popularity. Instead a variation, the diaphragm, was developed in 1880 and was called the Mensinga pessary after its inventor. This was a much larger rubber barrier, circular in shape and held in place over the cervix with a spring which pushed the cap tightly against the walls of the vagina. It became popularly known as the 'Dutch cap' because of its popularity with the early Dutch birth-control clinics.

Spermicides — substances which are toxic to sperms — were widely used, and the old-fashioned household solutions of lemon juice or vinegar were gradually discarded in favour of commercially prepared spermicidal jellies, the first of which appeared on the market in 1906.

Fumigation of the vagina or wiping it out with a sponge soaked in a spermicidal solution have been used for reasons of hygiene and to attempt contraception for many hundreds of years; but vaginal douching — rinsing out the vagina with a syringe — was claimed as the invention

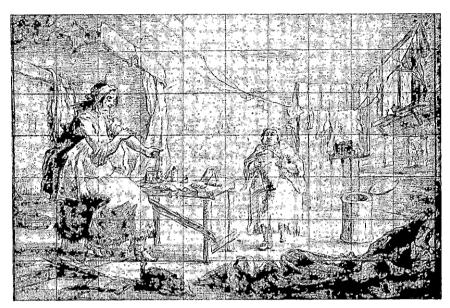

A harlot in her attic, surrounded by the tools of her trade – note the syringe and condoms washed, and hanging on the line. (Drawing by William Hogarth)

of the American Charles Knowlton in 1832. He asserted that it was harmless, cheap, would not cause sterility and did not impede coitus. It also kept control of contraception in the hands of women themselves. He recommended, without specifying strengths, solutions of alum, sulphate of zinc, sal eratus, vinegar or liquid choloride of soda.

The Wife's Handbook, a guide to contraception published in 1887, recommended an 'Irrigator':

> The Irrigator is a kind of can, holding about two pints, which is hung on the wall by the woman's side of the bed, at the height of some four feet or more above the level of her head. This can has a long india-rubber tube attached to a hole near its bottom, and at the mouth-piece end of the tube there is a little turn tap. Before getting in to bed the woman fills the can with a solution of alum and water, as recommended above, places a bed-pan and towel on a chair at the side of the bed; and after connection she has but to turn her back and slip the bed-pan under her; then she inserts the mouth-piece of the india-rubber tube into the vagina as far as possible, and the alum solution flows in and out again without causing wetting or trouble.[15]

Only the dedicated, one feels, would have bothered to use such a gruesome contraption.

Intra-uterine devices — to be placed in the uterus itself — were experimented with in the nineteenth century, but not properly developed until quite recently. For centuries similar devices had been used, but for a

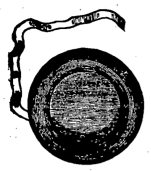
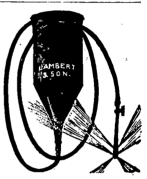
very long time they were thought to promote fertility rather than act as contraceptives. Tests began seriously on IUDs in the 1960s. The attractions of the device were plain: it was cheap, easy to insert, and once in place could be forgotten about, providing it did not cause side effects or was unwittingly expelled. While the device has undoubtedly served many millions of women well, there has been much concern about the risks of the IUD, including rejection, abdominal pain, heavy bleeding, an increased incidence of ectopic pregnancy and septic abortion. The IUD is not strictly speaking a contraceptive, for it does not prevent the coming together of egg and sperm; rather, by making the womb unreceptive, it prevents the implantation of the fertilised egg, which is expelled as an early miscarriage in the form of the monthly menses.

The biggest breakthrough in the search for an easy, effective and reasonably safe method of prevention of conception did not come until the middle of the present century with the development of an oral contraceptive agent, commonly known as 'the pill'. Recipes for oral contraceptives have been recorded for centuries; many had a herbal basis — willow tea, parsley and mint, lavender, marjoram, and fern roots such as 'barrenwort'. No serious work on contraception by suppression of ovulation could be undertaken, however, until the female reproductive cycle, the role of the hormones and the effective synthesis of oestrogen and progesterone had been effected, and none of this took place until the 1960s. When it came, its impact on the lives of millions of women was immeasurable.

The contraceptive story does not end with the pill: far from it. Research into new methods of contraception — some more satisfactory than the old ones, others plainly less so — continues apace. Implants which release tiny doses of hormones into the body over a period of up to five years are being developed; the 'morning after' pill brings on abortion by the ingestion of high doses of oestrogen; Depo-Provera is an injectable synthetic hormone (depot medroxyprogesterone acetate, or DMPA) which releases hormones into the blood stream over a period of three months or more. The disadvantage of DMPA is that, unlike the arm implants, now being developed, once injected it remains in the system until it finally works itself out. Unpleasant side effects, therefore — and there can be many — are irremediable.

Such rapid strides have been made in the field of contraception that it is easy to imagine that much more can be achieved; and technically that may be so. Yet public opinion now tends to safety rather than speed, and as we have become more conscious of the effects of filling our bodies with hormone additives, caution is inevitably the watchword.

In the field of male contraception *coitus interruptus*, the condom and vasectomy (sterilisation) are still the only widely available options. Research programmes are under way on male contraceptives — the notorious 'gossypol' from China is one — but there are problems with toxicity and loss of libido. Vasectomy, with the aid of modern microsurgical techniques, now has a higher chance of reversal, and new techniques such as the insertion of easily removable silicon plugs in the sperm tubes are being investigated, mainly in the East.

Most research is still concentrated on the interruption of the female reproductive cycle by hormonal methods or by new barrier protections. Vaginal rings which emit small amounts of hormone daily are being tested, and once-a-month post-coital pills are being researched. Tests are under way in Sweden on nasal sprays which contain tiny amounts of hormone that emit signals to the pituitary gland, prompting it to stop ovulation or sperm production. Work is continuing, too, on IUDs of improved design, some containing hormones which leach out into the body. Improved methods of female sterilisation are being looked at, one of which involves spraying liquid silicone into the fallopian tubes to block them; the plugs thus formed are designed for later removal if required. Spermicides are being constantly improved too, and should become both easier to use and potent for longer periods than products available today.

For those who rely on 'natural' methods of birth control, the paraphernalia of equipment to determine the 'safe' period becomes ever more extensive. Electronic thermometers and special calculators, saliva dipsticks or urine dipsticks to measure the presence or absence of certain chemicals in the urine are being developed; and an elaborate 'Ovutime Tackiness Rheometer' is available in the States — at great cost — to help determine changes in the nature of the vaginal secretion which can indicate ovulation. The Mucus or 'Billings' method was named after the Catholic doctor who described it in 1972.

One further major means of fertility control has also been developed — sterilisation. Modern techniques of sterilisation, both male and female, are now quick, simple, and even in some cases reversible. Removing the need for concern about contraception was, for many women, a godsend, although the more or less final nature of the operation has brought with it the need for responsible counselling and clear decision making. All in all, the available methods of contraception seem to be perpetually growing; while their acceptability, either physically or morally, remains a matter for debate.

The changing climate of opinion

A rudimentary knowledge of contraception has been passed down from generation to generation, just as knowledge about birthing and abortion were passed on. As the character of society changed, however, with a shift of population from rural community to industrial urban centre, so the age-old traditional patterns of communication were altered. As more and more people learned to read, 'book learning' was seen as more authoritative than information passed on through oral tradition.

It was hardly surprising, therefore, that in the nineteenth century there was a proliferation of written information and advice about contraception available to the population; and as knowledge became more public and the available contraceptive options grew, so there began a flurry of controversy which has only shifted in emphasis, not diminished, to the present day.

In 1823 Thomas Place, a Londoner, began to distribute a series of handbills, dubbed the 'Diabolical Handbills', addressed to 'The Married of Both Sexes'. The leaflets were dropped in quantity everywhere — on doorsteps, packed in boxes, handed out in the market place. They discussed points of birth control and recommended the use of sponge pessaries, and also the practice of *coitus interruptus*. Pessaries of wool or cotton were also in use at that time.

Two years later a man called Richard Carlisle published *Every Woman's Book: or What is Love?*[16] The book recommended both the sponge and *coitus interruptus* which, it was stated, 'is certainly effectual in all cases; but not so easily to be observed by all persons.'[17] The book included some gossipy information such as the story about the English

Duchess who 'never goes out to dinner without being prepared with a sponge'. French and Italian women, 'wear them fastened to their waists, and always have them at hand.'

In America, an awareness of the need for birth control was also growing at this period. In 1830 Robert Dale Owen, an expatriate Scotsman, published a book called *Moral Physiology*, in which he advocated *coitus interruptus* as a means of contraception. Following this, in 1833, was another book, *Fruits of Philosophy* by Charles Knowlton of Massachusetts (who claimed to have introduced the idea of vaginal douching). Other publications began to proliferate.

By the mid-nineteenth century, there was clearly a widespread interest in the whole question of birth control. The number of pamphlets increased, although there was always a great deal of controversy about their existence. One pamphlet, 'The Marriage Problem', printed and circulated privately by 'Oedipus', elicited a response from philosopher and humanitarian John Stuart Mill:

> February 19, 1868. I thank you for your pamphlet. Nothing can be more important than the purpose it has in view. About the expediency of putting it into circulation, in however quiet a manner, you are the best judge. My opinion is that the morality of the matter lies wholly between married people themselves and that such facts about which the pamphlet communicates ought to be made known to them by their medical advisers. But we are very far from that point at present, and in the meanwhile, everyone must act according to his own judgement of what is prudent and right.[18]

Certainly in America resistance to information about birth control was strong. In 1873 the New York Society for the Suppression of Vice was established, and the Comstock Law was passed, forbidding the distribution of contraceptive advice in the post.

In Britain by this time very many middle-class women were actively practising some form of contraception. This was a period when there was a general rise in the standard of living; and in those households where the income did not rise sufficiently to purchase the new wished-for comforts and luxuries, economies were looked for elsewhere. It became impossible both to have a large number of children and to give them all a good start in life, and one obvious answer was to have fewer children.

There were other factors at play too; a growing awareness, for instance, that sexual intercourse could be enjoyable if it did not always carry with it the risk of pregnancy. There was a greater interest in health, and a realisation that a large number of pregnancies was a tiring business. As society's notions of family life underwent a change, there was more pressure to give greater attention to children as individuals. Carlisle wrote in 1838:

> There is an ill-founded notion current, that to reproduce an
> unlimited number of children is beneficial to society. It is only a
> benefit to children to be produced when they can be made to be
> healthy and happy.[19]

It was a remark that women of the time began to appreciate; and by 1870
Dr Elizabeth Blackwell, the first American doctor, was able to go so far as
to say, 'I do not consider . . . that the object of marriage is to produce
children.'[20] Medical opinion stressed the need to restrict the number of
pregnancies in order to conserve the mother's health. A mother risked
her life in childbirth, and with every pregnancy the risk increased.

From 1877 when the birth rate in Britain was at its highest, suddenly it
began to drop, dramatically. It continued to drop until 1920. Literature
regarding birth control had been available — if only in a limited way —
from the early years of the century. Why, then, the sudden drop in the
1870s?

One factor may have been the notorious Bradlaugh-Besant trial of
1877-78. In the mid-1870s a Bristol bookseller, Peter Cook, was arrested.
He had been selling an illustrated version of *The Fruits of Philosophy* —
a book which had been available for some forty years. The reason for the
prosecution was that this particular bookseller had added a selection of
obscene pictures to the illustrated edition. He was prosecuted, and a light
sentence was imposed. Two members of the Free Thought Movement,
Annie Besant and Charles Bradlaugh, decided to publish the book
themselves, and they wrote to the police to tell them what they were
doing. Their idea was to force a trial in order to bring the matter to public
notice and to prove that there was no obscenity involved. The book, of
course, had been on sale continuously for some forty years, and there were
other books which also give illustrated accounts of contraception. The
verdict went against Bradlaugh and Besant but was quashed on appeal —
and the trial brought with it an enormous amount of publicity, bringing
the question of birth control to the forefront of the public awareness.

During the trial, sales of the notorious *Fruits of Philosophy* rocketed.
The gutter press cashed in on the whole affair. One pamphleteer,
William McCall, published *Malthusian Quackery* in which, among other
nasty capers, Breezy Bouncer (Mrs Besant) sang 'The Song of the Squirt'.
An anonymous poem published at this time ran:

> . . . after the coup,
> All the ladies need do,
> Is to jump out of bed on the spot.
> Fill the squirt to the brim,
> Pump it well up to her quim;
> And the kid trickles into the pot.[21]

There may, however, have been reasons other than the Bradlaugh-Besant
case for the decline in the birth rate. Marie Stopes points out that in 1876

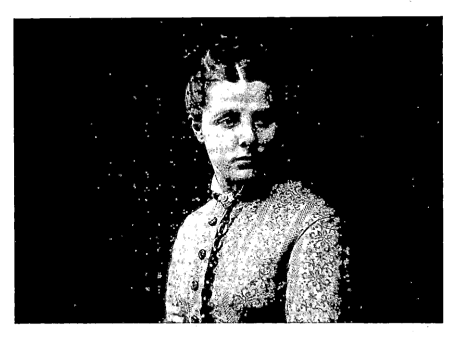

Annie Besant, one of the members of the Free Thought Movement who advocated birth control.

a new law was brought in that made registration of births compulsory. She suggests that a backlog of registrations — possibly several years overdue — could have given a false 'high' reading for the years 1876-7.

Birth control nevertheless remained controversial. Edward Truelove, a Free Thought publisher, was given a four-month prison sentence for publishing *Moral Physiology*, and in 1887 a Leeds doctor, Arthur Allbutt, was struck off the medical register for publishing a pamphlet called *The Wife's Handbook*, a leaflet which had been heavily subsidised by the new and steadily growing contraceptive industry.

The pressure for contraception, however, moved on. Significantly, the new contraceptive measures transferred the reponsibility for birth control into the hands of women themselves. Advertising pressed home the point that effective birth control brought health and well-being to women. This control over reproduction was the beginning of personal freedom for women, and they were not about to give up the fight. In 1878 the Malthusian League was set up by Annie Besant and C R Drysdale. Its aim was to press for the setting up of clinics to help women with their contraceptive needs. The first such clinic was established as an extension of her general practice in Holland in 1879 by Alletta Jacobs. Her own favourite method of birth control was the Mensinga vaginal diaphragm, or Dutch cap.

213

The Allbutt case had set back proper medical promotion of contraceptive devices in Britain, and Bradlaugh's Malthusian League was connected in the popular mind with atheism (of which Bradlaugh and Besant were both vocal adherents). The clergy spoke against contraception as an 'atheistical and materialistic doctrine'; so progress on the dissemination of information and the practice of contraception was slow at the turn of the century.

Gradually, however, the climate of opinion began to change. As writers began to explore the nature of sexual relationships in society one such book raised again the question of contraception:

> Apart from the pressure of population, it is time to be learning: (1) That annual child-bearing is still common, is cruelly exhaustive to maternal life, and this often in actual duration as well as quality; (2) That it is similarly injurious to the standard of offspring; and hence (3) That an interval of two years between births (some gynaecologists go so far as three) is due alike to mother and offspring.[22]

By the early years of this century, it was clear that the birth rate in the upper middle classes at least — and notably among doctors and the clergy — was considerably lower than among the working classes. In 1905 a committee of the Fabian Society was appointed to look into the birth rate and infant mortality statistics. The results, published in 1907, concluded that 'the decline in the birth rate is principally, if not entirely, the result of deliberate volition in the regulation of the married state'[23] — in other words, couples were practising some method of birth control.

Another publication had a profound influence on public opinion regarding contraception. *Sexual Ethics* by August Forel was translated into English in 1908. Forel pointed to the dangers of 'unlimited reproduction' the demands of which society would be unable to counter. As there were effective contraceptive controls available, he argued that:

> . . . the just and proper use of these methods must be described as ethically positive. Everything is moral which makes for the happiness and well-being of society: everything immoral which prejudices or endangers it.[24]

Forel's work, too, marked the beginning of an upsurge of interest in eugenics — 'the study of agencies under social control that may improve or impair the racial qualities of future generations, whether physically or mentally'.[25] It was argued that if only children who were planned for were born, there would be much more tenderness in the world. Many children did not mean fit children, and there were quite a number of doctors who argued for birth control in order to improve the standard of general health of the children who were born.

The tendency of the eugenists towards a doctrine of 'racial superiority' was, even then, noted and abhorred by many. But undoubtedly one factor that encouraged women to use contraceptive measures to limit the size of their families was the general improvement in medical care at this time. Now that they could reasonably expect their children to survive infancy and childhood and live to become adults, the need to produce a large family — in the hope that one or two of the infants would live to adulthood — had begun to pass.

The medical world at last began to show an interest in the matter of contraception. In 1912 Sir James Barr gave his support to birth control in his presidential address to the British Medical Association.[26] And, in America, where the dissemination of information about birth control was still forbidden, Dr A Jacobi, President of the American Medical Association, also endorsed contraception.[27]

The following year, 1913, saw the establishment in Britain of the National Birth Rate Commission under Bishop Boyd Carpenter. The report of the Commission was published in 1917, and a second report under the chairmanship of the Bishop of Birmingham was published in 1920. Both recognised the importance of some means of birth control.

In 1918 appeared *Married Love*, written by thirty-six-year-old Marie Stopes, a married virgin who had a mind to become the pioneer of contraception in Britain. It was well received, and in response to demand she published a supplement, *Wise Parenthood, a Book for Married People*.[28] As Stopes wrote in her book *Contraception, Theory, History and Practice*:

> The time was ripe, indeed over-ripe, for a consideration of the essential medical and physiological factors of contraception apart from a controversial cult of economics and party politics.[29]

The need to reach the working and illiterate classes with information about contraception became at once apparent, and Stopes — who strongly believed in the arguments of eugenists that the fertility of the poor should be severely curtailed — produced a basic leaflet with this in mind.[30] Margaret Llewelyn Davies' collection of letters, *Maternity, Letters from Working Women*, shows that even in the early years of the twentieth century, education among the working classes regarding contraception was minimal. Despite harsh economic circumstances, families were still very large, and the consequential suffering, both in terms of the mother's health and in material aspects, was very great. Llewelyn Davies, a compassionate observer, writes in her Introduction:

> The fact that the decline in the birth rate is greatest among the better-paid wage earners is often said to prove that a growing love of ease and luxury is causing a declining birth rate. The words 'ease' and 'luxury' are grotesque when applied to the lives of manual wage earners. The fact is that the industrial worker took the first seventy

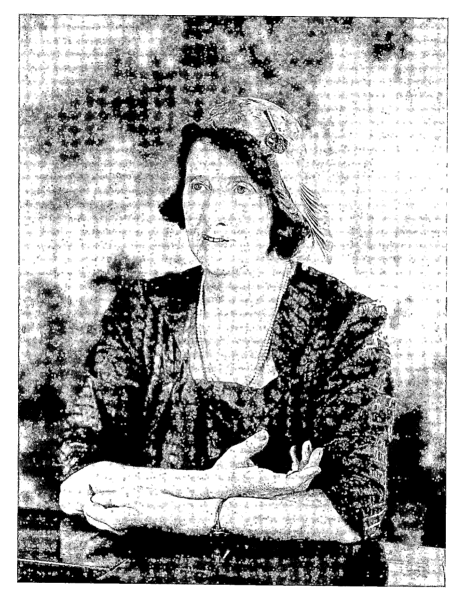

Marie Stopes wrote books of advice for young married couples, and opened a clinic to give free advice and contraceptive aids in 1921.

years of last century to learn that conditions such as described in these letters make a human and humane life impossible for mothers and children of large families.[31]

In 1921 Marie Stopes and her husband opened a small clinic in London, in the charge of a qualified midwife. Here not only free advice but free sponges, caps and suppositories were supplied. In order to lend weight to the work of the clinic, and in an attempt to open up the medical correspondence on the subject, Stopes held a meeting in the Queen's Hall in London, which was given tremendous support. The Women's Medical Federation held a series of meetings on contraception, and in August a correspondence was at last opened up in the pages of the *British Medical Journal*.[32] Gradually other clinics were opened, and Stopes founded the Society for Constructive Birth Control, which amalgamated in 1930 with other organisations to become the National Birth Control Association. In 1939 this became the Family Planning Association. In many other countries, too, efforts were being made to promote contraceptive education, although in France in 1920 a new legal ruling classed contraception with abortion and all matters concerning birth control became illegal. In America in 1919 the Voluntary Parenthood League was organised under the directorship of Mary Ware Dennett to promote the idea that parenthood should be a matter of choice and to bring about the repeal of the Comstock Law.

The driving force behind the struggle for contraception in America was Margaret Sanger. Sanger announced the first birth control clinic in the States in 1916 for the purpose of advising poor women; her activities were immediately stopped by the police. In 1917 she organised a monthly journal, *Birth Control Review*. In 1921 she founded the American Birth Control League, organised national conferences in Geneva, and founded the National Committee for Maternal Health.

The first birth clinic in America was the Birth Control Clinical Research Bureau in New York, established in 1923. The following year it was raided, and two women doctors and three nurses were arrested. The case against them was dismissed at their trial, and the incident only served to highlight the need for birth control information in the States. By 1931, there were many birth control clinics in America.

In 1946, after the end of the Second World War, Sweden proposed a meeting of birth control organisations in Stockholm, and as a result the International Committee on Planned Parenthood was set up by America, Britain, Holland and Sweden. In India in 1951 the first All-India Planning Conference was held, and in Bombay the following year that group met with the International Committee. From this meeting was born the International Planned Parenthood Federation, which now has members in some fifty-four nations.

Freedom of choice

For most women, the ability to have some degree of control over their own fertility is of critical importance in the organisation of their lives. In addition, the risks involved in using certain types of contraceptive — and there are undoubtedly risks involved with IUDs and hormonal aids — are in fact small when set against the risk of pregnancy and labour, or against the other option, abortion.

Seen overall, the impact of freely available contraception on the lives of women and their place in society has been immense. Nowhere is this demonstrated more clearly than in the changes that took place in western society following the advent of the pill. First and foremost the pill, combined with new techniques of sterilisation, alleviated the massive problem of multiparity. The grossly debilitating effects of bearing many children were solved simply and rapidly. To the go-ahead college woman of the early 1960s, the pill was a central symbol of freedom; and it coincided with a great surge of feminism. The pill and the women's movement went hand in hand.

> Since 1960, a woman is able to make a unilateral contraceptive decision without obtaining the co-operation of her partner. Until that point only men enjoyed such latitude. It is this autonomy in reproductive matters that is crucial to the development and manifestation of rational self interest. And without such rational self interest, freedom and responsibility are only a charade. In my judgement, the oral contraceptive has probably done more for equal rights for women than any other single phenomenon.[33]

In the early days of the pill, liberated young women were eager to obtain it: 'Long before its use as a contraceptive was officially authorised, we were wheedling the oestrogen pill out of our doctors,' wrote Germaine Greer.[34] Yet ironically, by the 1970s, a number of feminists were attacking the pill. Leading the attack was journalist Barbara Seaman, a medical writer from New York. Her book, *The Doctor's Case Against the Pill* stressed every negative aspect of oral contraception. Certainly early reports, many from Britain, underlined the fact that the pill was not without side effects, some of them dangerous.

Germaine Greer is one of the latest in a line of eager one-time pill users to change her tune: 'The problem with the pill is that we simply do not know what the deal is. What are we risking for what?'[35] Yet despite continued questioning of the long-term benefits and safety of the pill, it remains one of the most important and most widely used contraceptives today. And it has transformed the lives of not just western women but also of millions of women in underdeveloped nations for whom contraception had previously been impracticable.

> The diaphragm may be ideal for the motivated American women willing to use it, but it is totally unsuitable for the impoverished woman living in a hovel lacking running water, a toilet and privacy.[36]

218

For many such women, the touching of one's genitals is taboo, instruction by a male doctor would be unheard of, and the same strictures would apply to the insertion of an IUD, even assuming that trained workers were available to fit them.

For both demographic reasons (to control too huge an expansion in the world's population) and social reasons (for the general health and well-being of women), birth control is here to stay. Carl Djerassi, in his book *The Politics of Contraception,* asks:

> What should birth be like in the year 2001? In my opinion we need a contraceptive supermarket, that is, availability on a global scale of a repertoire of birth control devices and methods from which both men and women may choose, taking into consideration not only health factors but also their own cultural, religious and moral preferences.[37]

The problems of the development of new methods of birth control, Djerassi suggests, are not so much those of medical science, but of politics:

> Today's public opinion climate will have a profound effect on the future of contraception . . . for it is the politics of contraception rather than the science, that now plays a dominant role in shaping the future.[38]

In other words, the critical factor is not the ability of the researchers to provide methods of birth control suitable for mass use, but the willingness of governments to fund and implement programmes of birth control, and of popular acquiescence in such programmes.

Set against the desire of planners for demographic control is the opinion of some articulate, educated women in the west:

> It is our right to decide if and when we have children, on our own terms. We reject population control, which is about reducing numbers of births through a variety of persuasive and coercive policies; a major aspect of which is the provision of contraception and sterilisation programmes which are not necessarily based on women's needs. Population control, in all its forms, is essentially about controlling women.[39]

It is an argument that few family planners at an international level have cared to take into account; and attempts by internationally funded family planning organisations to control the birth rate of nations has been conspicuously unsuccessful. In India, vigorous mass male sterilisation programmes backed by Sanjay Gandhi resulted in over eight million sterilisations — still a small proportion of men in a population of over 711 million. In addition, there was a high incidence of post-operative complication, and 1,774 deaths. Aversion to the programme — and a fundamental distrust of all attempts by outsiders to impose birth control

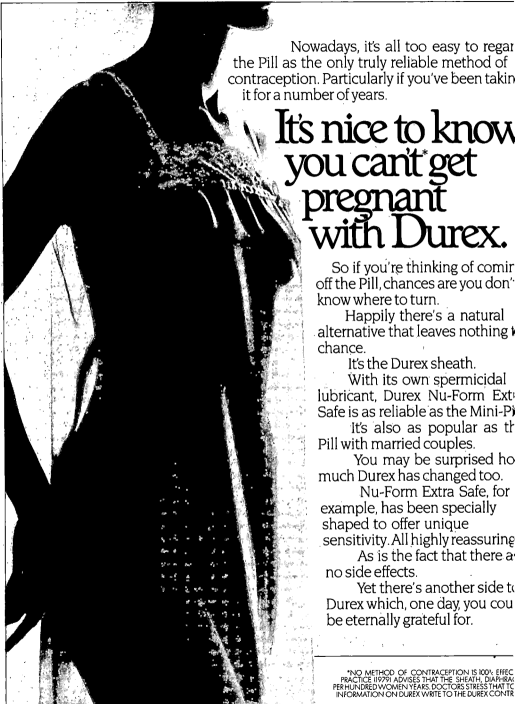

Nowadays, it's all too easy to regar
the Pill as the only truly reliable method of
contraception. Particularly if you've been takin
it for a number of years.

It's nice to know
you can't* get
pregnant
with Durex.

So if you're thinking of comir
off the Pill, chances are you don'·
know where to turn.

Happily there's a natural
alternative that leaves nothing w
chance.

It's the Durex sheath.

With its own spermicidal
lubricant, Durex Nu-Form Ext·
Safe is as reliable as the Mini-P·

It's also as popular as th
Pill with married couples.

You may be surprised ho·
much Durex has changed too.

Nu-Form Extra Safe, for
example, has been specially
shaped to offer unique
sensitivity. All highly reassuring

As is the fact that there a·
no side effects.

Yet there's another side t·
Durex which, one day, you cou
be eternally grateful for.

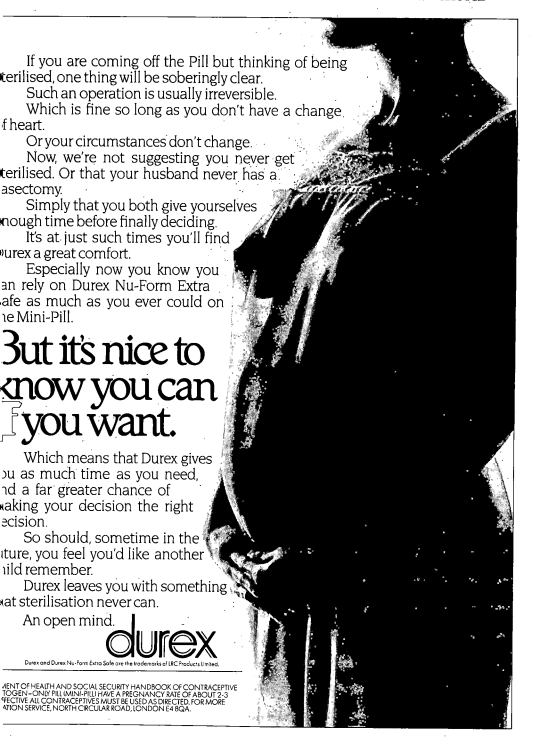

If you are coming off the Pill but thinking of being
sterilised, one thing will be soberingly clear.

Such an operation is usually irreversible.

Which is fine so long as you don't have a change
of heart.

Or your circumstances don't change.

Now, we're not suggesting you never get
sterilised. Or that your husband never has a
vasectomy.

Simply that you both give yourselves
enough time before finally deciding.

It's at just such times you'll find
Durex a great comfort.

Especially now you know you
can rely on Durex Nu-Form Extra
Safe as much as you ever could on
the Mini-Pill.

But it's nice to know you can if you want.

Which means that Durex gives
you as much time as you need,
and a far greater chance of
making your decision the right
decision.

So should, sometime in the
future, you feel you'd like another
child remember.

Durex leaves you with something
that sterilisation never can.

An open mind.

durex

programmes — was understandably strong. It must be remembered, too, that in a poor country like India children — potential breadwinners — are seen as a way to escape from perpetual poverty and hard work; and the infant mortality rate from infectious disease is high. Demographic programmers have frequently failed to take account of local culture, economics and psychology while drawing up their projection charts.

The imposition of birth control on nations or sections of nations is one thing; the desire by women to have an element of control over their own fertility is quite another. While the arguments over the subject continue, most are agreed on certain basic principles: to improve contraceptive aids that are available, to educate women about their own fertility, and to make the means of regulating that fertility available to all who wish it.

ABORTION — AS OLD AS LIFE

> Termination of pregnancy is one of the oldest and commonest forms of fertility control . . . The majority of women will resort to the operation in the face of religious and legal sanctions and will accept considerable pain, danger and expense to achieve their aims.[1]

> On a world-wide scale, abortion is one of the most important and widely-practised methods of fertility control among women and, whether we like it or not, will remain so for a long time.[2]

The fear of an unwanted pregnancy has always driven women to desperate measures. Mostly, abortion has been condemned — at an official level at any rate — and although it has been widely used as a means of controlling fertility for many thousands of years, morally, medically and legally abortion remains controversial.

Only since the 1970s has there been any medical literature on the subject of any depth or scope, and epidemiological, social, technical or demographic studies have been sparse. Modern literature reflects a relatively rapid change in attitude, and there is now a noticeably more sympathetic insight into the subject.

The forces that have driven women to seek abortion have always been as strong as they are diverse. In many cultures and many eras, giving birth outside marriage has been the signal for degradation and humiliation, the reason for a woman's being driven out of the family or community. Sometimes pregnancy is just the last straw, the final burden that will bring total misery to the poor, ill or overstrained mother of an already large family. In 1916 a working woman, worn down by poverty and previous pregnancies wrote,

> Now, is it possible under such circumstances for women to take care of themselves, during pregnancy, confinement, and after? Can we

wonder why so many women take drugs, hoping to get rid of the unwanted child, when they know so little regarding their own bodies, and have to work so hard to keep or help to keep the children they already have got?[3]

Ways and means

The ways in which women have attempted to procure abortion are many and often horrendous — scalding hot baths, falling down stairs, jumping off ladders, external binding, most of which would be as painful as they are likely to be ineffective. Massage, widely practised in many countries today, was well known in Europe for centuries; performed efficiently, it had a good chance of success. Certainly it was the most effective of all attempts to obtain abortion by external trauma.

Many early references to abortion now seem merely curiosities. Avicenna, who lived from 980-1037 in Persia, recommended that:

> Abortion may be produced, by those who abhor pregnancy, by prolonged baths and increased respiratory effort. The foetus is deprived of fresh air, and consequently dies. Abortion may also be induced by drugs, fasting, purgation, excessive coitus and massaging of cervical os.[4]

Folkloric remedies in the form of potions were innumerable. Many herbal concoctions were administered to speed labour, some with noticeable effect; thus, if they hastened labour by strengthening the contractions of the uterus, why should they not bring about uterine contractions in early pregnancy, and cause the expulsion of the newly conceived fetus? The principle was described in one mediaeval manuscript:

> Further, the things that cast out a dead child from the womb must be more powerful than those that assist in making childbirth easy.[5]

The idea was sound enough — though in this case the remedies might seem somewhat unorthodox:

> . . . 2 drachms of galbanum dissolved in goat's milk, so that the woman can easily take 2 or 3 ounces of the milk. [Or] make a suppository thus: take 2 drachms each of black olive oil, stavesacre, round birthwort, rosemary, marjoram, the seeds of laurel, the succulent part of colocynth, the gum ammoniac, and 1 drachm of bull's gall: reduce to powder, with the exception of the aromatic resin, dissolve the juice of artemesia, then mix with it all the other ingredients and make a suppository . . .[6]

Many were the plants associated with abortion. One of the most powerful was ergot. Derived from the fungus *Claviceps purpurea*, which grows as a little black protrusion on rye stalks, ergot had been in use for many centuries to help to strengthen uterine contractions during labour and to speed the delivery of the placenta. As an abortifacient, ergot is most effective in late pregnancy, and rarely before the fourth or fifth month.

Rue, *Ruta graviolens*, is another powerful abortifacient. In 1878, a case was reported of a young woman who had taken a concoction of

> ... three fresh roots of rue, about the size of a finger, sliced them up
> and boiled them in about a litre and a half of water, down to about
> three cupfulls, which she drank that evening, all at once.[7]

She had 'horrible stomach pain, vomiting and nausea', and she aborted two days later. Initially rue was thought to be simply a poison, but those doctors who thought that it acted as a powerful uterine stimulant were proved right by a researcher in 1941.[8]

Tansy, *Tanacetum vulgare*, was popular in some communities, notably in the United States, where tansy tea was a popular drink. Savin, *Juniperus sabina*, has been proved to have some stimulatory action on the uterine walls of animals, and it was used as an abortifacient in Roman times. Culpeper mentions the herb in his seventeenth-century book, *The Complete Herbal*: 'To describe a plant so well known is needless, it being in almost every garden.' Culpeper was well aware of the plant's properties: 'but inwardly it cannot be taken without manifest danger, particularly to pregnant women and those subject to flooding.' In *The Faery Queen* (1590), Spenser describes how the nurse 'had gathered Rew and Savine', and Dryden in *Juvenal* (1693) made no bones about its use: 'Help her make manslaughter, let her bleed, and never want for savix for her need.'

In eighteenth- and nineteenth-century Europe, the savin bush in the garden was a strong indication that the garden belonged to the local barber or midwife. In some areas the growing of savin was forbidden, and various botanic gardens found that they had to protect their rue. Yet the toxic effects of savin could be fatal — and not just to the fetus. Often the mother died too, frequently without previously aborting. Van de Warkle, an American obstetrician of the nineteenth century, tried savin on himself. The effects were not pleasant:

> A violent pain in the abdomen, vomiting and powerful cathartic
> action, the tenesmus, strangury, heat and burning in the stomach,
> bowels, rectum and anal region; intoxication, flushed face, severe
> headache ... salivation is often present. Its odour is clearly evident in
> the urine, which is increased in quantity and passed more frequently
> ... distressing hiccup is very generally present.[9]

To this were desperate women driven.

One of the main problems in using herbal potions to bring on an abortion was the question of dosage. The quantity of the herb used, how long it was boiled for, how much of the potion was drunk: all were critical in the final outcome. Nausea, vomiting, convulsions — these could be the total effect, or abortion could follow or death.

The alternative to herbal concoctions was direct intervention in the uterus itself. Insertion of sharp instruments into the womb has been a common method of abortion for centuries, and in some societies the use of a sharpened piece of bamboo or similar object is still common. In Britain in the early years of this century such instruments included crochet hooks, meat skewers, hairpins, goose quills, knitting needles, among others. Despite elementary attempts at sterilising these instruments by boiling, or by peeling the twigs, infection was common, and perforation of the uterine wall followed by haemorrhage and death was not unusual.

After Charles Goodyear perfected a means of vulcanising rubber in 1839, a new surgical instrument was developed — the rubber catheter, inside which a pointed needle was hidden. The catheter could be inserted into the womb until the conceptus was located, thus minimising the risk of injury to the vagina or uterine wall. By 1900, metal catheters were widely available in France, and one doctor wrote:

> It is recommended that the woman can best perform the operation unassisted, and I verily believe that the average Frenchwoman can locate her uterine os as certainly as she can touch the tip of her nose.[10]

She would dilate the cervix 'by rotary onward motion . . . until the sensation of rupture occurs and by the escape of bloody fluid proves the success of the operation'.[11]

The syringe was another method used for the termination of pregnancy in the nineteenth century. The syringe as a surgical instrument had existed for many hundreds of years, but the addition of a long nozzle made of rubber gave it the properties required for ejecting water at high force into the uterus itself. The resultant irritation of the uterine walls, or the actual dislodging of the placenta, brought on an abortion. In the mid-nineteenth century, such apparatus was commonly used by professional abortionists, but towards the end of the century it became widely available and was used by the woman herself.

The syringe, highly effective as a means of abortion, was not without risks. One obvious risk was that of infection if the apparatus was not properly sterilised — and particularly if the operation was performed by a less than meticulous midwife. Other risks were of damage to the vagina or uterus by the syringe, peritonitis caused by unclean water being forced into the peritoneum, or air bubbles passing into the veins and travelling to the heart or lungs. Despite the dangers, syringes were widely available in Europe at the end of the nineteenth and in the early twentieth century.

In England, the vaginal douche seems to have been more common than the uterine syringe, while douches sold in the United States may have been purely for contraceptive purposes. Solutions used for douching in the 1930s included lysol, carbolic soap, turpentine, iodine and water.

The procedure which followed the syringe as a means of procuring abortion, and which soon took over from it in terms of popularity and safety, was dilatation and catheter. The ability to induce the gradual stretching open of a tightly closed cervix was one of the useful medical advances of the nineteenth century. Once the cervix was opened sufficiently, a catheter could be inserted to irritate the uterine walls, and so induce abortion. Often merely opening the cervix would be sufficient. The procedure at first was used for genuine medical reasons — for example, early induction of labour in a woman with a contracted pelvis who could not be allowed to run full term.

Sometimes the bark of the American slippery elm tree was used to open the cervix. This was rolled tightly and slipped into the tight cervix; it expanded as it absorbed mucus. Later this procedure was superseded by the rubber bag, into which water was gradually pumped. Efficiency of the procedure was greater after four months of pregnancy. Dilators — a set of graduated instruments made of lead, pine or tin — were described in a work by Hippocrates in the fourth century BC. These instruments, used to achieve a progressive dilatation of the cervix, are essentially the same as dilators used today.

An instrument for scraping wounds clean was invented by a Frenchman in 1723; and the curette, as it was called, was adapted for cleaning the uterus by another Frenchman, Recamier, in 1842. Obstetricians James Young Simpson in Scotland, and Marion Sims in America, adapted the uterine curette for their own needs. Once the risks of infection had been reduced after the acceptance of aseptic techniques, the curette was used widely by doctors to scrape the inside of the womb. This could be for the removal of fungal growths, or to remove an incomplete delivery of the afterbirth or the after-effects of an incomplete abortion. Eventually the curette was used to perform the abortion itself, particularly in the early weeks of gestation.

As the nineteenth century wore on, women turned in ever greater numbers to the medical profession for help with termination of pregnancy; poorer women might turn to the midwife or herbalist, but those with money looked to the doctor. Women, especially urban women, rejected the old folkloric remedies in favour of new drugs in the form of pills. Many pills available in the drugstores and shops to 're-establish the menses' were based on laxatives, iron salts and alcohol, and had very little efficacy as abortifacients. Many of the old herbal drugs such as savin and rue were now difficult to obtain, and as a result were widely adulterated. Neither the female 'pills' nor these heavily adulterated herbal potions were likely to bring on the desired abortion. More drastic in their results were the new pills based on toxins such as lead, arsenic or phosphorous. Many could indeed bring about an abortion, but they were just as likely to kill the mother soon after the fetus. Pennyroyal, Epsom salts, silver-coated quinine pills, aloes, castor oil — few would produce any effect other than sickness. Other pills, more potent, might contain 'Hickey-pickey, bitter apple, bitter aloes, white diachylon (lead) — one pennyworth of each', one woman told the doctor after she had collapsed and aborted.[12]

The most widespread and possibly the most effective of the available abortifacients was lead. In the form of lead plaster, 'diachylon', it had been known since ancient times. Mixed with fats, it was sold in druggists as 'black stick', a compound used to hold bandages or used in place of plaster of paris to secure fractures. Bought easily, it could be broken into pills and swallowed. This type of lead pill — which could damage the nervous system and prove fatal in large doses — was popular with women in industrialised areas for forty years, and only fell off in popularity when sale of it in stick form was restricted.

At this time, in the mid-nineteenth century, ergot was still in use. In an article in the *British Medical Journal* one physician wrote that, 'he was in the habit of largely dispensing the medicine ergot . . . [and] was fully aware of its effects. He had known it to be given for three weeks.'[13] In the late nineteenth century quinine began to be imported from Java. Its properties for the alleviation of malaria were well known, and it soon became common knowledge that quinine had the effect of stimulating the uterus as well. As the popularity of ergot and lead as abortifacients declined, so that of quinine grew, and by the First World War it was one of the most commonly employed drugs for the termination of pregnancy. In small doses quinine did act as a uterine stimulant, but in large doses its effect was minimised, and it merely succeeded in paralysing the uterus.

Parsley, recommended for centuries as a contraceptive, had long been known, too, for its abortifacient properties. The difficulty lay in extracting the active ingredient in sufficient quantities to be effective. In 1847 two doctors from Paris, Homolle and Joret, managed to treat the seeds of parsley in such a way as to extract its essence, which they named apiol. The essence, designed originally as a treatment for malaria which might substitute for the very expensive quinine, proved in fact to have little effect on that disease — but it was soon noticed that it did have an effect on women whose periods had stopped. A new 'emmenogogue' had been found; and soon the drug, apiol, was widely prescribed for 'menstrual irregularity'.

In the early days of the present century, apiol was widely manufactured by a large number of drug companies. By the 1920s, it was sold over the counter at pharmacies to produce abortion, and by 1930 it was far and away the most popular of the means by which desperate women, suspecting that they were pregnant, attempted abortion. In America the drugs Ergapiol, a mixture of apiol, ergot, oil of savin and castor oil, and Apergol were available, though usually sold with discretion, under the counter.

Despite its widespread use, apiol was finally withdrawn from the open market in the 1950s on the grounds of safety, and was allowed to be dispensed on prescription only both in Britain and the States. Certainly, apiol did have a toxic effect in large doses, and there are a number of recorded deaths ascribed to the drug; but apiol, like quinine, was most effective as an abortifacient in small doses.

While pills and potions were being developed, though not necessarily improved, surgical methods relating to abortion most definitely were improving. In Edinburgh in 1863 Sir James Young Simpson described another method of 'menstrual regulation':

> I have made frequent use of a tube resembling in length and size a
> male catheter, with a large number of thickly set small orifices
> stretching along for about two inches from its extremity, and having
> an exhausting syringe adapted to its lower extremity, by which air
> could be withdrawn after it had been introduced into the cavity of the
> uterus. The use of this instrument is in some cases attended with
> striking results.[14]

This method of extraction, called 'dry-cupping', was one of the earliest recorded attempts at vacuum extraction. It took some time before it caught on. Despite its extensive use in Russia during the liberal period of the 1920s, vacuum extraction did not become a standard medical procedure in western Europe — particularly in Britain — until the late 1960s. Thereafter the technique, safe and easy to perform, became the most common method of termination of early pregnancy.

In 1961 a Californian, Harvey Karman, began to perform illegal abortions. He tried to perform vacuum extraction without having first to dilate the cervix. Suction curettes then used by the medical profession had only a single opening, and it had been found that when they were made from small-bore tubing the curette became rapidly blocked. Karman, using a flexible plastic tube of a much smaller bore, made two openings in it, and the results were encouraging. He was able to perform early abortions without the need to dilate the cervix, administer anaesthetic or encounter the problems of blocked tubes.

Induction of abortion at a later stage in pregnancy required different techniques. In the nineteenth century the introduction of a large rubber catheter after dilatation of the cervix was common, as was syringing the uterus with fluids such as medicated soaps, glucose or saline solutions, utus paste or urea. The surgical technique known as hysterotomy developed after it became possible to perform Caesarean section at full term. The operation involves the opening of the uterus through the abdominal wall, and the removal of fetus and placenta.

Generally speaking, the risk of complications from termination rise as the pregnancy proceeds. There can be problems from uterine perforation, haemorrhage, infection, pulmonary embolism (where a detached blood clot or air bubble travels up to the heart and round to the lungs, and can cause death), or death from a complication of anaesthesia. It is possible for dilatation of the cervix to cause later incompetence and make a further pregnancy difficult to carry to term. Infection caused by abortion can cause future sterility if not swiftly treated.

In the twentieth century new techniques for the termination of pregnancy were developed as the knowledge of hormones and the way they functioned increased. As early as the 1930s it was known that high doses of oestrogen administered within a few days of menstruation being overdue would bring on a period. If pituitrin was also given immediately after the oestrogen was withdrawn, the chance of restoration of menses increased.

Much research has been done on a group of proteins which were given the name prostaglandins (from the prostate, from which it was thought they derived). Nobel prizewinner Ulf von Euler pinpointed the action of these substances, found in human semen, on the uterus. Karmin in Uganda began to use prostaglandins to induce labour and in 1970 to induce abortion. The chemical synthesis of prostaglandins was achieved in 1969, making prostaglandin therapy much more readily accessible. Injection of prostaglandins directly into a vein, however, was found to produce too many unacceptable side effects; insertion into the vagina in the form of a pessary seemed to be better, producing 'only' headache, diarrhoea, cramps, dizziness, shivering and coughing. Such were these effects that the prostaglandins have not yet been produced for widespread use by women themselves, but are restricted to hospital terminations. In addition, they can produce incomplete abortion, which then requires surgical evacuation and further hospital treatment. As a second trimester abortifacient under hospital use, the prostaglandins are nevertheless less dangerous than most surgical techniques.

Research into abortion agents continues. In France a new pill, RU486, is being developed. It works by stopping the circulation of progesterone in the system. The uterus is thus unable to sustain any developing pregnancy, and abortion results. Trials of RU486 are being conducted in other countries.

Our bodies are our own

Attitudes to abortion have changed rapidly over the centuries and in different cultures. It was widely practised in ancient Greece and Rome, and seems to have been widely accepted especially if the mother's life or health could not be shown to be at risk. Christian morality dictated otherwise. Abortion was a direct contravention of the commandment 'Thou shalt not kill'. But if the formulation of Christian attitudes to abortion clearly concerned the question of the sanctity of human life, this may not have been the sole contributory factor:

> In studying the law relating to abortion it is natural to observe the contribution made by Christian doctrine, notably that concerning the sanctity of human life. However, while respecting the concept of 'revealed' religious truths, one may question whether this doctrine arose spontaneously and enquire whether there may have been social or communal factors which fashioned the religious attitude.[15]

Anthropological studies have indicated that in societies where there was a need to limit the size of the family, foeticide or infanticide was widely practised; and that, conversely, it is notable that 'a threat to tribal, national or racial survival by declining numbers could result in abortion becoming disfavoured and prohibited'.[16]

The early Christian Church certainly had a need to preserve and enlarge its strength — and that meant rearing more Christians. The evangelising spirit of the Crusades in the eleventh century, undertaken to enlarge Christian territory and add to the numbers of the faithful, also meant a commitment to bring forth new life (although it plainly did not preclude the killing off of large numbers of infidels). Thus abortion, and of course contraception, became forbidden by the Christian Church, and the attitude became absorbed into Christian doctrine.

In Britain, early abortion legislation was enacted under the ecclesiastical, not the civil courts, and it was not until 1803 that abortion law reached the statute books.

The burning question for philosophers and moralists, and for lawyers too, has always been — when does the fetus become human? Aristotle gave the dates as forty days after conception for a male fetus, ninety days after conception for a female fetus. As well as its odd gender discrepancy, the argument was purely philosophical, as there was no sure means of diagnosing the sex or establishing the precise date of conception. Some later theologians argued that abortion was criminal only if it took place after 'ensoulment'; and that the abortion of an 'unformed' fetus was acceptable. Many approved therapeutic abortion if the mother's life was at risk.

The literature appears to show a sharp increase in the number of abortions in the course of the nineteenth century, but the figures may be misleading. The fact is that with an increase in literacy and improvements in the keeping of official records, a higher incidence of abortion coming to official notice was recorded. It may also have been the case that in western Europe changes in medical knowledge, coupled with a growing awareness by women of their own bodies, meant changes in techniques of termination — techniques that were not always successful, so that a great many more cases of septic or incomplete abortion reached the hospitals for treatment. Women were now turning away from the old folkloric herbal remedies and putting their trust in newfangled devices — the rubber catheter, the douche or the syringe.

In the nineteenth century, too, a slow but steady rise in the standard of living was evident; women, aware of the limitations of their purses and increasingly conscious of the demands of childbearing and rearing on their own health and energy, set themselves deliberately to limit the size of their families through contraception and, if necessary, abortion. One writer in 1889 observed that:

> ... although the number of marriages is on the increase, the number
> of births to each couple is decreasing ... Instead of the number of
> cases of abortion undergoing a diminution an enormous increase is
> taking place, and this is all the more strange since our knowledge of
> maternal, paternal and foetal causes of abortion being investigated is
> steadily growing.[17]

Advertisements by abortionists were abundant, and usually only thinly veiled. One such, dated around 1868 ran:

> Mr__Consulting Accoucheur No.__ after many years devoted to the
> practise of midwifery in its most intricate forms, is enabled to afford
> the immediate relief in all cases of female irregularity however
> difficult. Early applications preferred.[18]

A series of reports in the *British Medical Journal* of 1868 looked closely at the very large industry of 'baby farming' and the domain of the illegal abortionist. Answering ambiguous advertisements like the one above, reporters would pose as worried husbands and visit the establishment in question. Often they were found to be neat and clean, with a piano in the parlour and 'uglier instruments in the cupboard'. The *Journal*'s own experiment of placing a false ambiguous advertisement drew 353 replies in one week. Clearly, these services were greatly in demand.

In America, too, women bent on achieving greater freedom from the demands and responsibilities of a large family turned with ever greater frequency to the abortionist: 'The ghastly crime of abortion has become a murderous trade in many of our large cities, tolerated, connived at and even protected by corrupt evil authorities,'[19] wrote one writer at the turn of the century. In 1871 Ely van de Warkle, addressing the Boston Obstetrical Society, declaimed that:

> ... the married woman who gives society the womanhood she ought
> to give humanity seeks the abortionist and by the outlay of a few
> dollars shirks the high destiny of a mother.[20]

231

In the late eighteenth and early nineteenth centuries, women relied heavily on over-the-counter drugs or self-induced abortion techniques. It was not until between the 1930s and the 1950s that demand for over-the-counter drugs fell very sharply; indeed, in this period they were hardly sold at all. Edward Shorter, in his book *A History of Women's Bodies*, ascribes the decline to the increasing medicalisation of women's health:

> For better or worse, women in the 1930s started placing responsibility for their medical fate in the hands of doctors and abandoning self help. Able to get instrumental abortions from doctors and paramedical abortionists with relative ease (compared with one hundred years previously), women stopped using drugs.[21]

In the hospitals, certainly, techniques for abortion were improving; and by the 1930s and 40s in Britain a small number of gynaecologists working within the hospital system began quietly to make their own interpretation of the law as it stood. In Scotland, Dugald Baird carried out an extensive programme of preventive medicine at his hospital in Aberdeen. Here he set up a birth control clinic, and implemented abortion and sterilisation programmes which had an outstanding success rate in lowering maternal mortality, still births and infant deaths. In his lecture 'A Fifth Freedom' which has become something of a classic, Baird cited his results as a justification for freeing women from what he called the 'tyranny' of excessive fertility.[22]

In deciding whether to terminate a pregnancy, Baird would take into account a great many factors such as the social environment of the mother, the number of previous pregnancies she had had, her general physical and emotional health, the health of her children, and the effect that fear of giving birth to a defective child might have on the mother — the kind of thinking that put him well ahead of his medical contemporaries. In his practice, Baird was aided by the differences in the law between the two nations. In Scotland, neither the Offences Against the Person Act (which governed prosecutions regarding abortion in England and Wales) nor the Infant Life (Preservation) Act applied; abortions carried out for 'reputable medical reasons' were seldom investigated.

In England, the 1930s saw the beginnings of pressure for reform, with many women's movements joining the call for liberal legislation. The Women's Co-operative Guild's Annual Conference in 1934 resolved overwhelmingly that:

> In view of the persistent high maternal death rate and the evils arising from the illegal practice of abortion, this Congress calls upon the Government to revise the abortion laws of 1861, thereby making abortion a legal operation that can be carried out under the same condition as any other operation.[23]

In 1936 the Abortion Law Reform Association, ALRA, was founded by a group of committed women under the chairmanship of Janet Chance. Her vice-chairman, Stella Browne, was a flamboyant figure with strong views:

> Abortion must be the key to a new world for women. It should be available for any woman, without insolent inquisitions or numerous financial charges, or tangles of red tape. For our bodies are our own.[24]

Attention to the law was focused by the case *R* v *Bourne* in 1938, when Aleck Bourne, a London gynaecologist, terminated the pregnancy of a fourteen-year-old-girl who had been raped by four soldiers. The case forced discussion for the first time on a point of law — when an abortion could be deemed to be deliberately and lawfully procured. The judge held that under certain circumstances an obstetric surgeon had not only the right but the duty to perform termination of pregnancy. Bourne was acquitted.

The advent of war forced the issue aside; and in the 1960s, backstreet abortion was still widespread:

> Among women taking overdoses of quinine because of unintended pregnancies, two had suffered permanent blindness,[25]

reported the *Telegraph* in 1965; and in the same year a letter to *The Times* stated:

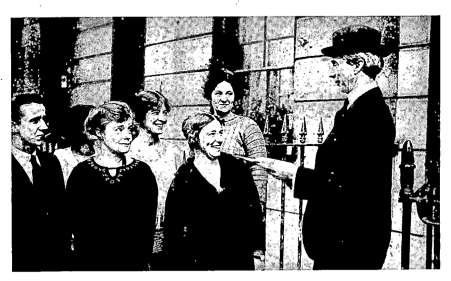

Stella Brown and Dora Russell, in the foreground, pioneers of ALRA, seen talking to Bertrand Russell.

> A teenage girl . . . had sought unqualified advice and was given a
> quantity of quinine to take. As a result of this, she had become blind,
> and it is unlikely that her sight will recover. The desired abortion
> was not produced — the reputation of quinine in this respect
> appears to be undeserved — and it remains to be seen whether the
> foetus has suffered the same fate as its mother.[26]

The one single event that served to trigger abortion reform was the
wave of birth deformities that followed in the wake of the thalidomide
tragedy. In America, Sherri Finkbane of Phoenix, Arizona, unable to
obtain a legal abortion in her home state, flew to Sweden to terminate her
pregnancy. The fetus was found to be severely deformed. In Britain,
abortion was at the time possible on the grounds of threat to the mother's
mental or physical health — but it did not include any provision for
consideration of possible deformity of the fetus. The debates that
preceded the reform legislation of October 1967 were long, complex and
impassioned. Once legislation was through, however, one important
effect was quickly apparent: the number of 'backstreet' abortions
resulting in infection, complications or even death, was very greatly
reduced. Women could now go to one of the newly set up pregnancy
counselling services, or they could go in the first instance to their own
GP. Opinion remained sharply polarised, but it did appear that:

> The volume of medical opposition to induced abortion lessened as
> more and more doctors came to face the viable reality of the problem
> of unwanted pregnancy among their patients.[27]

The three years following the 1967 Abortion Act in Britain saw a marked
increase in the number of abortions performed — highlighted, no doubt,
by the necessity, under the Act, of notifying all terminations. Thereafter,
the rise in the abortion rate levelled off while the birth rate began to
decline much more markedly. The inference must be that contraceptive
practice generally was improving. The mortality rate linked with
abortion fell too.[28]

The Lane Committee, reporting on the first four years of the Abortion
Act, concluded that 'by facilitating a greatly increased number of
abortions, the Act has relieved a vast amount of individual suffering', and
that instead of restrictive amendments to the Act, solutions —
professional and administrative — should be sought to all possible
problems. It was the opinion of the Committee that to seek restrictions

> when the number of unwanted pregnancies is increasing and before
> comprehensive services are available to all who need them would be
> to increase the sum of human suffering and ill health, and probably
> to drive more women to seek the squalid and dangerous help of the
> back-street abortionist.[29]

There have, in fact, been a number of attempts in Parliament to amend

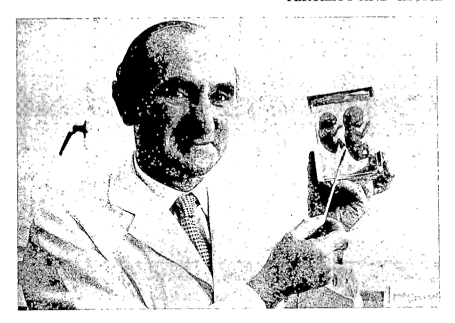

Professor Hugh McLaren strongly opposed abortion, and used to display a fetus in a bottle to emphasise his views on the rights of the unborn.

the 1967 Act, the most recent aimed at the reduction of the number of weeks' gestation before which abortion may be permitted. The reason for this move has been the rapid advance of medical expertise, which has enabled younger and younger infants to be 'viable':

> It is difficult to see why all the medical stops should be pulled out to save a scrap of humanity who is wanted by his parents while an aborted foetus that might live is an embarrassment to everyone; where is the essential difference?[30]

It is a debate yet to be concluded.

In America, and in most western European countries, there has been some degree of legal provision for abortion; indeed, according to one source, 36 per cent of the world's population can now obtain abortion on request and another 24 per cent for social reasons. A further 16 per cent may obtain abortion for medical or humanitarian reasons, and 13 per cent have restricted access to abortion. Only 8 per cent of women live in a country where abortion is completely illegal.[31]

Few women would regard abortion as a first choice of birth control, but the fact remains that:

> On a world-wide scale, abortion is one of the most important and widely practised methods of fertility control among women and, whether we like it or not, will remain so for a long time.[32]

235

For centuries, desperate women have had to resort to termination of pregnancy by whatever means possible. Thus the option for responsible termination of pregnancy is regarded by a large section of the population as indeed the 'fifth freedom'.

INFERTILITY — A NEW TECHNOLOGY

> *Never.* That verdict of 'never', though softly spoken, leaves the woman shaking, empty, her face too naked, her private grief too unconcealed.[1]

> The people who have least need of issue . . . are the only people who have access to the technological means of reversing their infertility.[2]

> . . . Lesley was speechless, but her expression was so moving, her look so eloquent that words were unnecessary. She cradled the infant and then managed to whisper. 'Thank you for my baby. Thank you'[3]

The body is a brilliantly designed piece of machinery; intricate and complex in the extreme. And like any complex piece of machinery, it performs well if it is taken care of. But always there remains the possibility that something might go wrong.

In respect of fertility, the efficiency of the mechanisms controlling conception is usually such that most women who wish to avoid becoming pregnant must take positive measures to interfere in some way with the reproductive cycle — in other words, they must use some method of contraception. For others — a very small number overall — the problem is the reverse. Some snag in the body's machinery — either the woman's or her partner's — causes an inefficiency in the reproductive system, and conception becomes less likely, or impossible.

Emotionally, infertility can cause deep heartache; the desire to reproduce is a very strong biological urge. When a couple wish to start a family, prolonged inability to conceive can be devastating.

In the past, before the physiology of human reproduction was properly understood, the likelihood was that it would be the woman who was 'blamed' for the lack of issue unless there were some obvious problem in her partner such as disease, disability or impotence. And whatever the cause, or whoever was 'to blame', there was in any case virtually nothing that could be done to remedy the situation. Adopting a child was certainly one option; and before abortion became widely available, there were more babies available for adoption.

The importance of fertility is central to many societies and cultures:

> . . . the notion of fertility underlies many human ethical systems, including our own, although in a residual and fragmented form. The management of fertility is an essential aspect of maturity . . .[4]

In the western world, infertility is not only a problem which seems to be increasing constantly — estimates currently suggest that one in six couples today are infertile — but it also 'has an important impact on a couple's personal relations and consequently on their mental and physical health and may influence their social and economic status'.[5]

The causes of infertility are many. Adverse influences include radioactivity — from the horrendous effects of atomic explosion, witnessed after Hiroshima and Nagasaki, to the generally rising levels of radioactive fall-out in the atmosphere — as well as the more common problems caused by disease and malnutrition or the effects of drug addiction. Stress, a symptom of modern society, can lead to cessation of ovulation or some other upset of the delicate reproductive mechanism. Sexually transmitted diseases, widely prevalent in the sexually permissive society of the west today, can be a major source of infertility: gonorrhoea, in particular, presents a problem as it is primarily asymptomatic — that is, a woman may contract the disease without ever being aware of it. Gonorrhoea attacks the fallopian tubes, and can have the effect of totally blocking them. Often it is only when a woman who has contracted the disease in this form attempts to conceive that the problem becomes apparent.

The ability to tackle the problem of infertility is very much a modern phenomenon. Only this century, and really only since the 1930s, has the human reproductive cycle been understood — and even now, many of the intricate secrets of fertility remain to be uncovered. The exact role of the oviduct, for example, is still a mystery: 'After more than half a century of clinical interest in female infertility, we are unable to assess accurately a single physiological function of the fallopian tubes.'[6] Research into menstruation together with greater understanding of the hormones, the study of embryology and the growing sophistication of technical apparatus have, however, tempted scientists and medical researchers into the field of human reproduction in an unprecedented way. Treatment of sexually transmitted disease, too, has to some extent been made possible by the advent of antibiotics.

To push forward the boundaries of knowledge of the reproductive system seems a logical part of humans' general determination to understand the way in which our bodies work; and once we understand, the temptation to interfere seems irresistible. Faced with a woman who is inconsolable about her inability to conceive, it would be a hard gynaecologist who would not desire to help if the means were available. Yet viewed statistically the situation may seem odd: why strive so ardently to increase the population when there is such a massive need to restrict the general trends of population growth?

Germaine Greer, in her book *Sex and Destiny*, has pointed out the irony that

> ... the people who have least need of issue (in the absence of land which must be worked by the younger members of the family or kinship systems to advance), who have unlimited possibilities of satisfaction in the field of commerce, political power and intellectual activity, are the only people who have access to the technological means of reversing their infertility.[7]

Whatever the demographers may say, whatever the statistic sheets show, the fact is that infertility causes great grief and heartache. And many couples are prepared to tackle the problem in whatever way they can, whatever the cost. Today, the possibilities for the reversal of infertility are good, and they are increasing.

The treatment of infertility has risen as a sub-discipline of obstetrics remarkably rapidly in the last decade or two. The work of men like Patrick Steptoe and Robert Edwards in Britain in the field of *in vitro* fertilisation (where the egg is fertilised outside the female body — literally 'in glass') has become legendary.

To produce a baby by the delicate and complex method of retrieving the eggs from the ovary, fertilising them *in vitro* and reimplanting them — 'test tube' fertilisation — is the ultimate option for the infertile couple. It may be possible that preliminary investigations would reveal some problem quite simply rectified. Where the cause of infertility is tubal blockage, however, the problem of treatment is great. It is often not possible to repair blocked or damaged tubes, and there is therefore no chance that the egg will ever descend through the tube to be available for fertilisation. In that case, and where the sperm count of the male or the motility of the sperms is considered severely abnormal, the only answer — and it is a very recent development in terms of medical history — is to retrieve an egg or eggs from the ovary itself, fertilise it outside the womb, then attempt to reimplant the fertilised egg in the woman's uterus.

The work on the test tube baby programme was largely undertaken in Britain by two men — Robert Edwards and Patrick Steptoe. Edwards, an embryologist, describes his first view of an egg, ripening in a culture fluid, outside the body:

> ... when I did examine the final oocyte I felt as much excitement as I had ever experienced in all my life. Excitement beyond belief. At twenty-eight hours the chromosomes were just beginning their march through the centre of the egg. Fine, clear, absolutely visible, a sight to reward all my past efforts. A living, ripening, human egg, unbombarded by any hormones, beginning its programme ... There, in one egg ... lay the whole secret of the human programme ...[8]

Edwards' need for human ova to experiment on led him eventually to meet and to start a collaboration with Patrick Steptoe, a consultant gynaecologist based in Oldham, Lancashire. Steptoe had long been practising a diagnostic technique with a new instrument called a

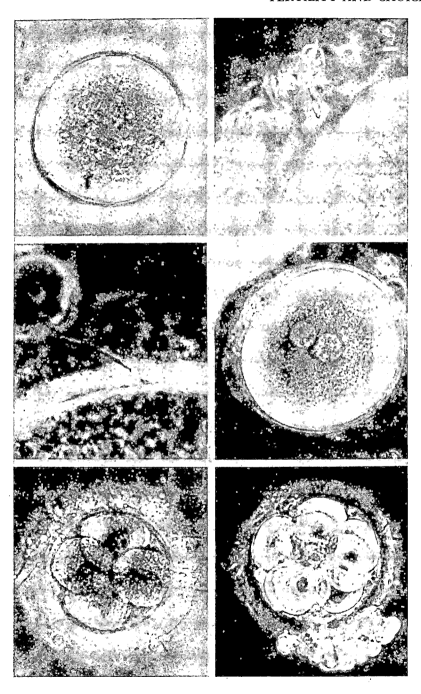

The early stages of embryo development – the division of the cells.

laparoscope. The laparoscope was a kind of telescope which had an eye piece at one end and a lens at the other, permitting a direct view of the organs of the body. In Britain, gynaecologists had been slow to accept the instrument, but Steptoe perfected his technique, using new and more refined instruments, and was soon using the laparoscope for diagnostic purposes as well as for sterilisation. It was an easy matter to remove samples of sperms from recent intercourse from the fallopian tubes and ova from the ovaries — material which could be of the greatest use to Edwards in his research.

Edwards'. attempt to fertilise ova *in vitro* proved fruitful; and in February 1969 the results were published in *Nature*. The first test-tube baby was still some way off, but the door was open.

The ethical dilemma

Very early in his work, Robert Edwards had realised that *in vitro* fertilisation would stir a hotbed of debate. Opposition came not least from within the medical profession. In 1971, an application made by Edwards and Steptoe for funding of a prolonged research programme was turned down:

> ... the Council ... had serious doubts about ethical aspects of the proposed investigations in humans, especially those relating to the implantation in women of oocytes fertilised *in vitro* which were considered premature in view of the lack of preliminary studies on primates and the present deficiency of detailed knowledge of the possible hazards involved.[9]

Indeed, from the time that news of successful *in vitro* fertilisation was made public Edwards and Steptoe had to combat criticism from many quarters. Edwards himself never doubted the validity or the morality of his work: 'I never belittled the strength of feelings that some have had about our work on early human embryos,' he wrote in his book, *A Matter of Life*;[10] but plainly the work excited him as a scientist, and as a compassionate man:

> ... if we were successful, and we fully expected to become successful eventually, we would open up the world of human embryology. There would be new approaches in medicine. We would bring hope to thousands upon thousands of infertile women and there might be all kinds of other benefits to human kind.[11]

From the beginning, the work on the fertilisation of human ova outside the womb was to provoke questions of ethics. Once the first 'test tube baby' had been delivered, on 25 July 1978, the storm well and truly broke loose. Plainly, the possibilities open to medical science were

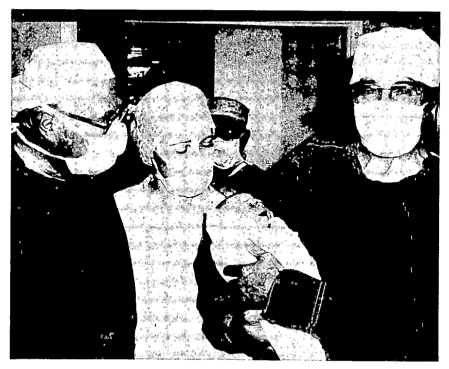

The birth of the first test tube baby, Louise Brown, 25 July 1978.

growing, and fast. To debate the ethics was clearly necessary — 'necessary because the fact that we *can* do something does not mean that we *ought* to do it'.[12] More particularly, the debate was necessary not merely for the fact that *in vitro* fertilisation had been achieved, but because:

> the new techniques of being able to initiate life outside the body bring with them other possibilities as well. They bring with them the possibility of manipulating the genetic structure of this budding human life; and the prospect of genetic engineering and cloning.[13]

Leaving aside for the moment the questions of genetic engineering and cloning, and looking at the processes involved in the *in vitro* programme itself, it is plain that here, too, there are many questions raised.

> Next morning the temptation to replace the blastocysts into the mother on the spot was very strong, and I have often wondered what might have happened had we succumbed. They belonged not to us but to the husband and wife who had donated their eggs and spermatozoa.
> 'What are we going to do with them?' asked Patrick.
> 'We're going to flatten them for chromosomes,' I replied.[14]

Edwards was fully conscious that some embryos would not be replaced in the womb of the mother but would be used for experimentation. Later, surplus embryos might be frozen — they were, in the words of one of the Australian *in vitro* team, a 'by-product' of the *in vitro* project.

Most of the debate about the ethics of embryo experimentation centres on the question of the moral status of the embryo itself, in exactly the same way as the ongoing debate about abortion calls into question the status of the fetus:

> It is hardly an adequate response to this concern for a medical scientist to point out that a two-cell embryo 'cannot be seen by the naked eye'. If it is judged to be human, which seems reasonable and, still more, if it is to be regarded as a person, which is more debatable, then it enters into the arena of moral responsibility just as surely and to the same extent as other human beings or persons whom, for geographical or other reasons, the naked eye does not see.[15]

The complexities of the moral and ethical situation surrounding the extraction of ova from a woman and fertilisation of that ova *in vitro* are immense. Who owns the embryos? If the sperm and ova are donated by a husband and wife, it is normally presumed that they are in agreement about their participation in the programme, and have given 'informed consent' to experimentation. But what if the eggs are donated by the wife and the sperm by a donor? Or what if they are transferred to another uterus, not that of the wife? The permutations are endless, but the resulting ethical considerations are enormous. The legal situation, too, has become deeply convoluted. What was to happen, for example, to the frozen embryos of a couple who were simultaneously killed in a car crash? And what if the child conceived as a result of *in vitro* fertilisation was deformed? Who would be held responsible?

Similar questions are raised by the practice of surrogate motherhood. Surrogate — substitute — motherhood is the process whereby a woman agrees to bear a child on behalf of a woman who for some reason is unwilling or unable to bear it herself. The advantages of this to the couple wishing to have the child is that the baby will at least be half their own — the father having donated the sperm. Indeed, the child could be genetically wholly their own if both sperm and ova were donated. Again, the whole question raises complex issues. In Britain, the notion of 'handing over a baby' on the basis of a paid contract seems to generate a great measure of repugnance; in the possibly more commercially based American society, there is certainly not the same degree of abhorrence to the notion of paid surrogacy, and agencies to control and deal in surrogate motherhood are not uncommon.

Again, the legal issues can become very complicated. What, for example, if the surrogate, having entered into a contract to bear the child, and having accepted money for that purpose, decides after the baby is born that she will not hand over the child? Is the contract legally enforceable? Who is the 'natural' mother of the baby — to whom, in most cases, custody would normally be given?

It was with a view to examining the 'social, ethical and legal implications of recent, and potential developments in the field of human assisted reproduction'[16] that the Government in Britain appointed a Commission, chaired by Dame Mary Warnock, to report into Human Fertilisation and Embryology. The Committee, popularly known as the Warnock Committee, presented its report in July 1984.

Faced with problems of immense complexity, the Warnock Committee had its work cut out; and, ultimately, it was not able to reach unanimous conclusions on a number of issues, notably the questions of surrogacy and embryo research. Regarding surrogate motherhood, it was the overall recommendation of the Committee that agencies for the promotion of surrogacy should be made illegal, and that persons aiding surrogacy should be made criminally responsible. As regards embryo research, it was the overall recommendation of the Committee that no research should be carried out on fertilised eggs *in vitro* after the fourteenth day.

It was the intention of the Government that the findings of the Warnock Committee should be given time for discussion and debate before any recommendations regarding changes in the law governing embryo research, *in vitro* fertilisation, surrogate motherhood and so on were drafted. The questions raised were new, and it was felt that a certain time was required for assimilation and understanding of the complex issues involved. The position changed dramatically, however, when a Private Member's Bill was brought before the House by Enoch Powell early in 1985. The Unborn Children (Protection) Bill attracted widespread support, and threatened an end to the future of embryo research. Mr Powell, speaking in the House of Commons on 15 February 1985, said:

> When I first read the Warnock report I had a sense of revulsion and repugnance, deep and instinctive, towards the proposition that a thing, however it may be defined, of which the sole purpose or object is that it may be a human life, should be subjected to experiment and its destruction for the purpose of the acquisition of knowledge . . . I ask the House to . . . decide that . . . the moral, human and social cost of that information being obtained in a way that outrages the instincts of so many is too great a price to pay.[17]

The Bill received its second reading. Plainly, whatever the medical viewpoint, and despite popular support for a programme of research for *in vitro* fertilisation, popular public opinion was against embryo research. Yet the two go inextricably hand in hand, and a ban on embryo research effectively spells the end of research into *in vitro* fertilisation. What the future of such a programme might be in Britain is not at present clear.

243

Fertility and research — the future

Understanding the development of the embryo — possible only through extensive research and study — will lead, so the scientists claim, to a greater ability to prevent miscarriage, improve fertility, facilitate research into new methods of contraception and, possibly, to the ability to understand and therefore help to avoid genetic disorders which can run into thousands of kinds.

The enormity of the implications of embryology and genetic research in general, however, have possibly led to a general panic in the popular mind; surrogacy, *in vitro* fertilisation and further, genetic engineering (the control of hereditary defects by the elimination of certain genes), cloning (asexual reproduction by division of cells), ectogenesis (development outside the body) and hybridisation (the interbreeding of different species, for example man and monkey) — these are areas which many people find unacceptable even to contemplate.

One woman undergoing *in vitro* treatment wrote lucidly about the anguish she had experienced at her inability to have children, and of her feelings about the treatment in general:

> Scientists should not have to make ultimate ethical decisions about the morality of the work they do. ... It is ordinary people like us with intelligence and education who must use that power and tell the scientists how to help us and why we want to be helped. We must make the final decisions regarding the morality of what we are doing. . . . The couples who need to make choices about their fertility now are getting on with the job. They have no time to sit and think, 'Is IVF the right way to go?' For many, the only question they have ever asked is 'Do we want a baby?'[18]

Public debate about the whole question of human assisted fertility will and should go on; but for the infertile couple, the way forward is quite clear. No demographic demonstration, no theological debate, no searching querying of ethics will fundamentally affect their decision. All debate, for them, has long since been superseded by the overwhelming need to procreate.

REVALUATIONS

. . . joy rather than sorrow, hope rather than gloom, life rather than death.[1]

There is no doubt about it — childbirth has come a long way since the days of the formidable 'granny' midwife or the barber-surgeon with his grotesque array of hooks and knives; since severe blood loss after birth inevitably spelt death, or infection could set in with dire consequences. While women — even women with ready access to the best of hospital facilities — do still die in birth, fear of death is no longer the natural companion to childbirth.

Once the major problems associated with delivery — blood loss, sepsis and pain relief — had been solved, researchers began to turn their attention to other fields of research. Rontgen's discovery of X-rays at the turn of the century was developed as an aid to obstetric diagnosis, though by 1956 Alice Stewart in Oxford had inferred a link between X-rays and infant leukaemia. Then in the 1960s Ian Donald in Glasgow, seizing his inspiration from the ultrasonic echo systems he had seen used during the war for the detection of enemy submarines, developed ultrasound for use in obstetrics. Even more recently, another type of body scanning has been developed — nuclear magnetic resonance imaging (NMR).[2]

X-rays, ultrasound, NMR imaging — these are all methods developed for 'looking into the womb'. They are not the only means of assessing the well-being of the fetus which are at the modern obstetrician's disposal; the fetoscope, improved following the refinement of fibreoptics, allows the obstetrician direct visualisation of the fetus and its surroundings. And amniocentesis — the drawing off of a sample of fluid from the amniotic sac surrounding the baby — can provide diverse information. Cells cultured from the fluid can determine the sex of the unborn infant, and can provide the geneticist with valuable data about disorders the unborn baby might have inherited. The work of David Brock and Roger Sutcliffe in Edinburgh in 1972 on alphafetaprotein (AFP) provided a means of testing the fluid for the presence of neural tube defects, anencephaly (where the brain fails to develop) or spina bifida (literally, divided spine). Indeed, Brock and Sutcliffe took their work a step further and began to administer AFP tests on blood samples taken from pregnant women at routine antenatal visits. An AFP peak indicated a high level of risk, and the woman could then be referred for amniocentesis or further testing.

Work on the glands and the discovery of hormones brought further advances in medical knowledge which came to be applied to gynaecology and obstetrics. The understanding of the activity of the anterior pituitary gland and the discovery of the hormones oestrogen and progesterone led to many major developments. One of the earliest was the evolution of reliable methods of pregnancy testing; the Ascheim-Zondek method of injecting mice with a sample of urine was used from the late 1920s, but has been superseded by immunological or immunoassay methods of pregnancy testing.

The phenomenon of menstruation has been surrounded through the ages and widely across cultures with reverence, suspicion or aversion, and was often surrounded with taboos. Little scientific work was done until the isolation of oestrogen from the human ovarian follicle in 1923, but once an understanding of the mechanisms of menstruation and human fertility had been reached, many further fields of research opened up.

Perhaps the most far-reaching development to come from this area of research was the oral contraceptive pill devised by Gregory Pincus and his team in America. Following the synthesis of the hormone progesterone in 1943, and modifications to the molecule to increase its efficacy by Ehrenstein the following year, Pincus found a point in the female cycle that was 'attackable'; 'the pill' suppressed ovulation — and with no egg to fertilise, conception became impossible.

Apart from giving millions of women — some of them for the first time ever — the chance to control their own fertility, the new ability to space the bearing of children in a controlled way brought with it an enormous improvement in the general health of women. The debilitating effects of multiparity could become a thing of the past.

An appreciation of the effect of drugs on the developing fetus has been another step forward for twentieth-century medicine. Little serious research on the effect of drug ingestion during pregnancy was done before the thalidomide tragedy of 1961. It was understood that drugs given to the mother during labour could affect the baby, but the impact of drugs during pregnancy, particularly early pregnancy, had simply not been systematically investigated. Thalidomide had been thought to be perfectly safe; research on rats had demonstrated no adverse side effects, even when taken during gestation. A large number of deformed children were, however, born to women who had taken thalidomide, and finally the connection was admitted and the drug withdrawn. Thalidomide, it was noted, had very specific effects on the fetus which depended on the exact date of ingestion.

Teratology — originally the study of animal or vegetable monstrosities — had begun around the 1930s, when research was focused on the lower mammals. Now the scope of teratology has widened, and scientists are concerned with the tendency of a drug to induce abnormalities when administered during pregnancy; research covers behavioural and intellectual development as well as physical growth. Since the 1960s considerable work has been done on teratogens. The work involves the study of a very large number of pregnancies, and records are maintained on the complications of pregnancy, the occurrence stillbirths and spontaneous abortion, as well as on birth defects. The field is a complex one, and results difficult to prove definitively; the effects of a drug will vary considerably according to the amount taken, the stage of pregnancy at which it is consumed, whether the condition for which the drug is taken itself affected the pregnancy, and so on. The awareness of how drugs can affect the developing fetus is important, for the range of drugs available today is considerable, from the seriously addictive hallucinogenic or 'hard' drugs like heroin through to antinauseants, over-the-counter painkillers, nicotine, caffeine and alcohol.

Addiction to, or excessive consumption of, any one of these agents can be the cause of damage to the developing fetus. This was first discovered in relation to alcohol addiction which, at its most extreme, can produce in babies a condition known as 'fetal alcohol syndrome'. Symptoms of the syndrome may be seen even in babies born to mothers whose drinking has been relatively moderate. Another commonly consumed drug which can affect the development of the unborn fetus is nicotine. Nicotine constricts the blood vessels, and this in turn can affect the supply of blood to the uterus, and hence to the placenta, thus causing a reduction in the amount of oxygen to the fetus. It can also cross the placenta and affect the development of the fetal organs. Research has shown that the incidence of spontaneous abortion among smokers is twice as high as that in non-smokers — and the risk increases with the number of cigarettes smoked.

Normally when drugs are prescribed for pregnant women they are thoroughly tested beforehand. There have, however, been exceptions. From the 1940s to 60s the drug Diethylstilboestrol was prescribed to many thousands of pregnant women to prevent miscarriage, even though research carried out in the 1950s demonstrated that the drug did not do this. In the early 1970s, a link was discovered between young women with vaginal cancer and the ingestion during pregnancy of this drug by their mothers. Debendox, prescribed as an antinauseant during pregnancy, was another drug thought for many years to be quite harmless to the fetus. Recently a number of mothers in America have attempted to win compensation for the damage which they claim has been caused to their children through their ingestion of the drug. While the manufacturers of Debendox have withdrawn the drug from the market under pressure, the controversy continues, along with claims and counterclaims for the drug's safety.

Medical research has taught us more and more about our bodies and what happens to them during menstruation, in pregnancy and in labour. Doctors have been given the means to diagnose potential problems at ever earlier stages of pregnancy, and have been concerned to use these means to reduce the rate of mortality and morbidity of mothers and babies throughout the birth process. The result of this concern in turn led to the belief that the only safe place for women was under their care, and in hospital. For a decade or more, throughout the 1960s birth in British hospitals took on an increasingly regimented nature, and institutional routines were imposed on women willy nilly. Women, themselves concerned to improve the chances of their own and their babies' survival, at first accepted such treatment unquestioningly. In addition, the hospital represented for many women a new kind of freedom — freedom from the heavy chores of running a home and the confines and responsibilities that represented.

From the 1960s, however, some women began to query the wisdom of this dependence on hospital care and the associated dominance of the male obstetrical profession. They began to feel that the doctor's point of view was not necessarily right — or at least, that it took account of only one side of the question of childbirth. There was another — the quality of the experience of the birth, and the right of the mother to be treated as a person of intelligence and awareness, not as a production-line machine.

This dissatisfaction on the part of women coincided with a gradually growing awareness of values other than the technological ones which have taken an increasing hold this century. In all areas of progress, a period of evaluation generally follows initial euphoria; and older wisdom is often reassessed. Regarding childbirth, the pendulum certainly began to swing in this manner.

The relearning process can be seen, for example, in the pressure to return to postures used by primitive tribes: sitting, squatting, kneeling:

> A priori, the supine position is probably the worst in mechanical terms, since it makes no use of the force of gravity.... Any position which the woman finds most comfortable is obviously the most efficient. However, while some women choose to squat, to kneel or to sit in a special chair, others prefer to lie down. Three centuries of custom will not be eradicated in a few years.[3]

While Michel Odent's 'three centuries' is undoubtedly an exaggeration, the point is that there is a trend away from the imposition of any specific position, in favour of the personal choice of the mother. The birthing chair, referred to above, fell out of favour in the 1840s, supposedly because of the fear it engendered in women; interestingly, a hundred years on, it has made a reappearance. Michel Odent himself sees the chair as an imposition by the obstetrician:

> We do have a wooden obstetrical chair, but I don't want to emphasise it, because obstetricians will only remember the chair in their search for tne perfect device for birthing. Doing that, they overlook the whole concept of giving the mother total freedom.[4]

Yet the birthing chair does represent a further 'choice' and a compromise between the primitive postures which are no longer habitually used in western society and the more recently favoured supine position. A return to older remedies is witnessed, further, in the increasing use of massage, creams and lotions both in preparation for and during birth. In respect of episiotomy, for example, certain literature recommends the practice of perineal massage with almond oil or other emollients:

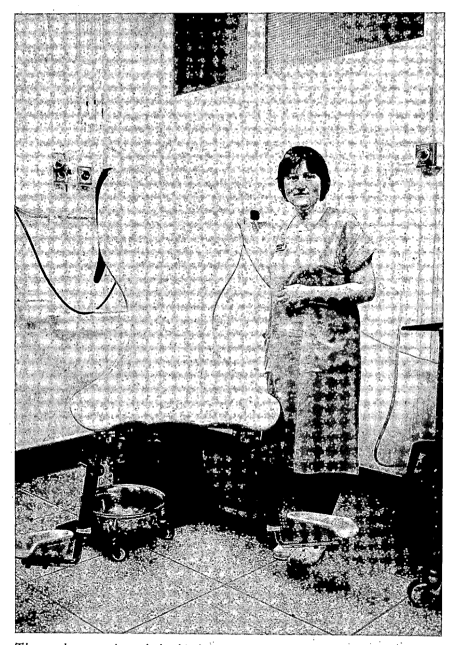

The modern version of the birthing chair, which has seen a resurgence in popularity.

> He massaged the area until the cream (in this case cocoa butter) was
> completely worked in, which typically took four or five minutes....
> After only one week, there was a noticeable increase in flexibility and
> strechiness.[5]

More dramatically, there has been a marked trend towards the rejection of the use of drugs in childbirth, both for the purposes of induction and for pain relief. In the late nineteenth century women, desperate to move on from centuries of childbirth agony, exerted great pressure on their doctors to administer pain-relieving drugs. They little understood — no one fully understood — what effect these drugs might have on them or their babies.

This whole area of drug administration is a complex one. One must remember that the women of the nineteenth century who clamoured for pain relief were, on average, considerably less healthy and well fed than women of today; and, in addition, were more likely to have many pregnancies, which had an increasingly debilitating effect on their frame. Now, a hundred years on, more women are aware of the possible adverse effects of such medication and many wish to experience the birth of their child with complete consciousness. Yet education about the birth process, about fear, tension and pain, has not by any means removed the need of most women for the alleviation of pain during childbirth. The contemporary 'natural childbirth' movement has done much to balance the march of technology; but, conversely, it has tended to make many women feel inadequate when actually confronted with the reality of pain:

> Women tell their husbands not to allow them to change their minds
> and demand drugs in a moment of weakness. They lock themselves
> into a childbirth of great pain because they have been told it is 'best'
> for them and their baby.[6]

The need for women to re-examine old wisdom may have stemmed in part, from the loss of the traditional support systems which surrounded her in the past. In our increasingly mobile society, there has been a gradual erosion of old forms of community care. Fewer mothers can rely on an extended family and the evolution of the nuclear family with its tendency to self-sufficiency has led to increasing isolation.

In terms of pregnancy and childbirth, the importance of continuity of care has been well demonstrated, and should form in part some compensation for this loss of community backup. Women do not like being seen by one doctor at an antenatal clinic on one visit, a different one on each subsequent visit, to be delivered finally by a complete stranger. The problem of continuity of care has not been fully tackled in this country, although there is a wide awareness of the need.

It is becoming clear that the routines imposed by many hospitals have undergone considerable change in the last five or more years. This may be seen as a response by the profession to a persistently presented need on the part of women for care which is more than purely medical. No longer do most hospitals in Britain now administer routine enemas or shave pubic hair. Fathers are widely admitted into the delivery room — although, interestingly, some birth movements now claim that birth should once more be exclusively a woman's affair and that the male in the birthing room can be no more than a distracting influence. The prone position is no longer rigidly insisted on — in many hospitals, the mother will be allowed to take any position she chooses during the birth, except in cases of complication. Postnatal bonding has been recognised as desirable, and no longer is the newborn baby whisked away for bathing and weighing.

Despite these elements of change, ongoing research is continuing to make available technological discoveries to 'aid' the birth process. Indeed, the scope has become so enormous that the Royal College of Obstetricians and Gynaecologists is already recommending that obstetricians begin to develop their own subspecialities within their field — divided roughly into 'reproductive' medicine, including gynaecological endocrinology, infertility and all the developing techniques attached to that area and 'fetal' medicine, which would involve the recognition and management of the high-risk fetus, and close involvement with other medical disciplines including 'medical genetics, perinatal pathology, biochemistry, bio-engineering and neonatal paediatrics'.[7]

Perhaps the most revolutionary development of the last decade with regard to obstetrics has been the development of neonatal paediatrics. Now it is possible to keep alive babies of twenty-eight weeks — or even younger — by means of ventilators and intensive care, with a very precise knowledge of the needs of the infant; and this in turn fundamentally affects decision-making by the obstetrician. Now, if need be, he or she can perform a section at twenty-eight weeks, in the knowledge that mother and baby may thus have a better chance of survival. But as with all other aspects of modern medicine, the possibilities raise fundamental questions: when to give up? How much should a baby be made to undergo? And what of the emotional reaction of the parents to all that is happening to their child?

The rapid escalation of technology in the field of birth can, in addition, conjure up curious pictures:

> There appears to be no limit to the mechanical invasion of the delivery room. The American T J Kriewall (*University of Michigan News*, March 1975) has actually put the finishing touches to a prototype 'dilatometer' which suppresses vaginal touch, records cervical dilation and translates into computer language the energy expended by the labouring woman with the help of a small magnet fixed to one side of the cervix and a small magnet feeler attached to the opposite side!

> Will the obstetrician of tomorrow be sitting in front of a computer
> terminal screen?[8]

Ivan Illich, in his book *Medical Nemesis*, proposed that as a society we
are becoming increasingly a slave to our tools.[9] In childbirth, such 'tools'
are coming under increasing scrutiny and women, more aware than ever
before of their bodies and the way in which they function, now allow little
in the way of 'development' to pass unquestioned. There is, after all,
another side to the question, as Iain Chalmers wrote in 1978:

> If one lesson emerges from the British debate on obstetric practice is
> that there is a need to establish the effects of interventions in
> perinatal medicine, then the other is that a maternity service which
> loses touch with the feelings and expectations of its clients will not
> . meet its needs.[10]

The last hundred years have brought changes to childbirth which are
staggering in the enormity of their impact. The implications of modern
technology are complex, extending far beyond the practicalities of 'can
we?' 'can't we?' into 'should we?' or 'shouldn't we?' This technology has
put the birth process increasingly firmly into the hands of the specialist,
the obstetrician; and there are some who will argue that that in itself is
almost too high a price to pay for safety. To others, the reduction in
mortality and morbidity speaks for itself.

For a woman, the dilemmas which face her are very different from
those of a hundred years ago: not, 'will I die?' but 'what will the quality of
my baby's life be?' Not, 'why can I not bear children?' but 'can embryo
research be considered ethical?' In a way, the future holds a different sort
of fear — the vision of a society in which the individual wishes of women
are subordinated to those which another sector of society perceives to be
to her benefit, a society in which midwife has given way to machine,
technology has quenched humanity.

It is for us to look at that vision, and to reject it; to draw from medical
progress the best it has to offer, and to mould that into a birth that can
truly give 'joy rather than sorrow, hope rather than gloom, life rather
than death'.

FOOTNOTES

EVE'S LEGACY

Women in society

1 Quoted in Carolly Erickson, *The Medieval Vision* (Oxford University Press, 1976), p. 189.
2 For a more detailed study of the development of views on women see: C Erickson, op. cit., chapter 8; Angela M Lucas, *Women in the Middle Ages* (Harvester Press Ltd., 1983), chapters 1, 2 and 8; Eileen Power, *Medieval Women* (Cambridge University Press, 1975); Evelyn Acworth, *The New Matriarchy* (Victor Gollancz, 1965).
3 *The Holy Bible*, Revised Standard Version (Oxford, 1952-71): Ecclesiastes 7:28.
4 *Hali Meidenhead*, ed. T J Furnival (Early English Text Society, o.s. 18, 1922; reprint, 1969), 524-6.
5 *Holy Bible*, op. cit., I Timothy, 2:15.
6 Geoffrey Chaucer, *The Complete Works*, ed. F N Robinson (Oxford, 1957), p. 259.
7 Geoffrey Chaucer, *The Wife of Bath's Prologue and Tale*, ed. J Winny (Cambridge, 1965), 149-53.
8 G R Owst, *Literature and Pulpit in Medieval England* (Oxford 1961), p. 377.
9 D W Robertson, *A Preface to Chaucer. Studies in Medieval Perceptions* (Princeton, University Press, 1962), quoted in Erickson, op. cit., pp. 202-3.
10 L Gautier, *La Chevalerie* (Paris, 1884), p. 350.

What was birth like?

1 Florence E F Barnes, ed., *Ambulatory Maternal Health Care* (n.p. American Public Health Association: Committee on Maternal Health Care, 1978), p. 18.
2 Suzanne Arms, *Immaculate Deception: A New Look at Women and Childbirth in America* (Boston: Houghton Mifflin, 1975), p. 8.
3 Edward Shorter, *History of Women's Bodies* (Basic Books, 1982), pp. 48-9.
4 Franz Strohmayr, *Versuch einer physisch-medicinischen Topographie von ... St Pölten* (Vienna, 1813), pp. 117-18.

5   Alexander Hamilton, *Treatise on Midwifery* (Edinburgh, 1781).
6   Christian Pfeufer, 'Über das Verhalten der Schwangeren... auf dem Lande', *Jahrbuch der Staatsarzneikunde*, 3 (1810), p. 49.
7   For examples of indulgence: R Westphalen, *Petit dictionnaire des traditions populaires Messines* (Metz, 1934), p. 327; Freddy Sarg, *La Naissance en Alsace* (Strasbourg: Oberlin, 1974), pp. 12-13; Yvonne Verdier, *Façons de dire, façons de faire* (Paris: Gallimard, 1979), pp. 49-52.
8   Shorter, op. cit., pp. 20-2.
9   Pfeufer, op. cit., p. 49.
10 R. Beaudry, 'Alimentation et population rurale en Périgord au XVIIIe siècle', *Annales de démographie historique* (1976), pp. 52-3.
11 Westphalen, op. cit., p. 328.
12 Aloys Winterling, *Die baüerliche Lebens-und Sittengemeinschaft der hohen Rhön* (Cologne, 1939), p. 88.
13 Quoted in Rosalind Mitchell, *Virgins and Viragoes* (Collins, 1982), p. 109.
14 Charles White, *Treatise on the Management of Pregnancy and Lying-in Women, and the Means of Curing, but more especially of Preventing the Principal Disorders to which they are liable* (1772).
15 Bernard Christian Faust, *Gedanken über Hebammen und Hebammenanstalten auf dem Lande* (Frankfurt, 1784), p. 31.
16 Thomas Raynalde, *The Byrth of Mankynd* (1954).
17 Quoted in R P Finney, *The Story of Motherhood* (New York: Liveright, 1937), p. 155.
18 Quoted in Beryl Rowland, *Medieval Woman's Guide to Health* (Ohio: Kent State University Press, 1981), p. 34.
19 Ibid. p. 34.
20 Nicholas Culpepper, *Compleat and Experienc'd Midwife in Two Parts* (3rd ed., London, 1718), pp. 55-6.
21 Sir Walter Scott, *Letters on Demonology and Witchcraft* (New York: Citadel Press, 1970), p. 126.
22 G Henslow, *Medical Works of the Fourteenth Century* (Chapman & Hill, 1899), p. 32.
23 Percival Willughby, *Observations in Midwifery* (1863; reprint East Ardsley: S R Publishers, 1972), p. 14.
24 Quoted in T Cianfrani, *A Short History of Obstetrics and Gynaecology* (Illinois: Charles C Thomas, 1960), p. 262.
25 Charles D. Meigs, *Obstetrics*, 5th ed. (Philadelphia, 1867), p. 329.
26 Jean Paul Stucky, *Der Gebärstuhl: Die Gründe für sein Verschwinden im deutschen Sprachbereich* (Zurich: Juris, 1965), p. 37.
27 F Ramsbotham, *The Principle and Practices of Obstetrics, Medicine and Surgery* (London, 1841), pp. 195-6.
28 Scottish Record Office, Leven and Melville Papers GD 26/401/29.
29 Scottish Record Office, Campbell of Barcaldine Papers GD 170/2034/9.
30 Moritz Gerhard Thilenius, *Kurzer Unterricht für die Hebammen und Wöchnerinnen auf dem lande* (Kassel, 1769), 66, pp. 6-7.

Hazards of childbirth

1 Cotton Mather, 'Hour of Travail and Trouble', quoted in Richard & Dorothy Wertz, *Lying-in* (New York: The Free Press, 1977), p. 21.

2 Scottish Record Office Leven and Melville Papers GD 26/13/466.

3 Josceline 'Mother's Legacy', British Library Add. Mss. 27 467: Reynolds, *Learned Lady*, p.29.

4 Ibid.

5 Entry in 1813 quoted in Carl N Degler, *At Odds: Women and the Family in America from the Revolution to the Present* (Oxford University Press, 1970), p. 59.

6 Women's Co-op Guild, *Maternity: Letters from Working Women* (1915), p. 166.

7 Doris Haire, 'The Cultural Warping of Childbirth' in John Ehrenreich, ed., *The Cultural Crisis of Modern Medicine* (New York: Monthly Review Press, 1978), p. 194.

8 Edward Shorter, *History of Women's Bodies* (Basic Books, 1982), pp. 71-2.

9 Ibid., p. 75.

10 Margaret Hagood, *Mothers of the South* (1939; reprint New York: Norton, 1977), p. 115.

11 Jacques Dupaquier, *La Population rurale du Bassin Parisien à l'époque de Louis XIV* (Paris: Editions de l'école des hautes études en sciences sociales, 1979), p. 364 for data on a sample of nine villages in the seventeenth and eighteenth centuries.

12 Shorter, op. cit., deals with the whole incidence of rickets in great detail, pp. 22-8.

13 Quoted in Rosalind Marshall, *Virgins and Viragoes* (Collins, 1983), p. 116.

14 Percival Willughby, *Observations in Midwifery* (1863: reprint East Ardsley: S R Publishers, 1972), p. 16.

15 William Smellie, *Treatise on the Theory and Practice of Midwifery* (London, 1752), p. 82.

16 Shorter, op. cit., p. 28.

17 W R Wilde, 'A Short Account of the Superstitions and Popular Practices relating to Midwifery . . . in Ireland', *Monthly Journal of Medical Science*, NS 35 (1849), pp. 721-2.

18 Rudolf Temesváry, *Volksbräuche und Aberglauben in der Geburtshilfe . . . in Ungarn* (Leipzig, 1900), p. 54.

19 G Lammert, *Volksmedizin und medizinischer Aberglaube in Bayern* (Würzburg, 1896), p. 166.

20 Anon., *Kurzgefasste Gedanken von dem Verderbeten Zustande des Hebammen* (Lubeck, 1752), pp. 7-8.

21 Willughby, op. cit., p. 164.

22 Louis Baudelocque, cited in Johann F Osidander, *Bemerkungen über die französische Geburtshülfe* (Hanover, 1813), p. 160.

23 Lisbeth Burger, *Vierzig Jahre Storchentante: Aus dem Tagebuch einer Hebamme* (Breslau, 1936), p. 20-1.

24 Guillaume Mauquest de la Motte, *Traité complet des accouchemens* (1715; reprint Leiden, 1729), p. 282.

25   E Pelkonen, *Über volkstümliche Geburtshilfe in Finnland* (Helsinki, 1931), p. 292.
26   Francois Mauriceau, *Observations sur la grossesse et l'accouchement* (Paris, 1694), p. 3.
27   Shorter, op. cit., p. 95.
28   Notice, *AJO*, 7, (1874-5), p. 164.
29   See Shorter, op. cit., pp. 106-9 and the whole of chapter six for a full study of infection in women following birth.
30   Alphonse Leroy, *Essai sur l'histoire naturelle de la grossesse et de l'accouchement* (Geneva, 1787), p. 146.
31   D Berry Hart & A H Freeland Barbour, *Manual of Gynaecology* (Edinburgh, 1886), p. 164.
32   Shorter, op. cit., p. 109.
33   Jacques-René Tenon, *Mémoires sur Les Hopitaux de Paris* (Paris, 1788), p. 222, 239-40, 269.
34   Ibid.

Rising expectations

1   Rosalind Marshall, *Virgins and Viragoes* (Collins, 1983), p. 279.
2   Patricia Branca, *The Silent Sisterhood* (Croom Helm, 1975), see chapters 4 and 5.
3   Robert T Conquest, *Letters to a Mother, for the Management of Herself and her Children in Health and Disease: Embracing the Subjects of Pregnancy, Childbirth* ... (London, 1848), p. 11.
4   Edward Shorter, *History of Women's Bodies* (New York: Basic Books, 1982), p. 30.
5   W D Buck, MD, 'Extract from the address of the president of the New Hampshire Medical Society for 1866', *New York Medical Journal*, 5 (August, 1867), pp. 464-5.
6   *The Magazine of Domestic Economy*, Vol II (March, 1844), p. 391.
7   Quoted in J M Munro Kerr (ed), *Historical Review of Obstetrics and Gynaecology* 1800-1950 (1954), p. 146.
8   M Ryan, *Philosophy of Marriage* ... (1837), p. 202.
9   Charles D Meigs, MD, *Females and Their Diseases* (Philadelphia, 1848, p. 19.
10   Robert Brudnell Carter, *On the Pathology and Treatment of Hysteria* (London, 1853), p. 69.
11   Quoted in W Radcliffe, *Milestones in Midwifery* (Bristol, 1967), pp. 71-2.
12   Ibid.
13   Ann Douglas Wood, 'The Fashionable Diseases', *Journal of Inter-disciplinary History*, 4 (1973), p. 36; Georg H Napheys, *The Physical Life of Woman* (Philadelphia, 1880), p. 169.
14   James Young Simpson, *An Account of a New Anaesthetic Agent as a substitute for Sulphuric Ether in Surgery and Midwifery* (1848), quoted in Radcliffe, op. cit., p. 84.
15   Munro Kerr, op. cit., p. 226.

16 'Why Not? A Book for Every Woman: A Woman's View', *Boston Medical and Surgical Journal*, 75, No. 14 (Nov. 1, 1866), pp. 273-6.
17 Quoted in Myrtle Simpson, *Simpson the Obstetrician* (Victor Gollanz, 1972), p. 143.
18 Ibid., p. 140.
19 Ibid., p. 140.
20 Annual Report of The Registrar General; Vol. XVII, (1884-85) pp. 1 xxii, 2. 63; Vol. xx iii-1 (1895) p. 193.

WHO HELPED DELIVER?

The traditional midwife

1 Elseluise Haberling, *Beitrage zur Geschichte der Hebammenstandes: Der Hebammenstand in Deutschland vom seinen Augangen bis zum Dreissigjahrigen Krieg* (Berlin, 1940), p. 29.
2 Edward Shorter, *History of Women's Bodies* (New York: Basic Books, 1982), p. 38.
3 Haberling, op. cit., p. 90.
4 Ibid., pp. 36-7.
5 J Sprenger and H Institoris, *Malleus Maleficarum*, trans. H. Summers (London, 1928), pp. 268, 66, 100, 140-1; M Hofler, *Volksmedizin und Abergaube in Oberbayerns, Gegenwart und Vergangenheit* (Munich, 1888), p. 199.
6 W Gubalke, *Hebammen im Wandel der Zeit* (Hanover, 1964), p. 16.
7 Beryl Rowlandson, *Medieval Woman's Guide to Health* (Ohio: Kent State University Press, 1981), p. 11.
8 Ibid., p. 167.
9 In German: *Der Swangern Frauen und Hebammen Rosengarten*.
10 Quoted in Myrtle Simpson, *Simpson the Obstetrician* (Victor Gollancz, 1972), p. 53.
11 Quoted in W Radcliffe, *Milestones in Midwifery* (Bristol, 1967) p. 22.
12 Quoted in Adrienne Rich, *Of Woman Born* (Virago, 1977), p. 141. Translated for her by Richard Howard.
13 Shorter, op. cit., pp. 44-5.
14 Dietrich Tutzke, 'Über statistische Untersuchungen als Beitrag zur Geschichte des Hebammenwesens im ausgehenden 18 Jahrhundert', *Centaurus*, 4 (1956), p. 354.
15 C F Senff, *Über Vervollkommnung der Geburtshülfe* (Halle, 1812) p. 41.
16 J B Gebel, *Aktenstücke die Möglichkeit der ganzlichen Blattern-ausrottung . . . betreffend* (Breslau, 1802), pp. 130-1.
17 J H Wigand *Beyträge zur . . . Gebürtshulfe* (Hamburg, 1800), p. 82.
18 Alöis Noth, *Die Hebammenordnungen des XVIII. Jahrhunderts* (Wurzburg: med. diss., 1931), p. 17.
19 Shorter, op. cit., p. 61.
20 Anne Amable Augier du Fot, '*Catéchisme sur l'art des accouchemens pour les sages-femmes de la campagne* (Soissons, 1775), p. xi.

Midwifery in Britain

1 J H Aveling, *English Midwives: Their History and Prospects* (London, 1872) pp. 31-4.
2 Antonia Fraser, *The Weaker Vessel* (Weidenfeld & Nicolson, 1984), p. 442.
3 *Diary of Samuel Pepys*, ed. with compendium and index by Robert Latham and William Matthews, 11 vols (1970-8), 11, p. 110.
4 Fraser, op. cit., p. 443-40.
5 Jane Sharp, *The Compleat Midwife's Companion* (4th edn, 1725), preface.
6 S Cutter & H Viets, *A Short History of Midwifery* (1964), p. 49.
7 Quoted in Walter Radcliffe, *Milestones in Midwifery* (Bristol, 1967), p. 9.
8 Jane Sharp, *The Midwive's Book, or the whole art of Midwifery Discovered* (1671), p. 3.
9 R P Finney, *The Story of Motherhood* (New York: Liveright, 1937) p. 101.
10 Elizabeth Nihell, *A Treatise on the Art of Midwifery: Setting Forth Various Abuses Therein, Especially as to the Practice with Instruments* (London, 1760), p. 167 n.
11 H R Spencer, *The History of British Midwifery 1650-1800* (London, 1927), p. 73.
12 Nihell, op. cit., p. 71.
13 John Maubray, *The Female Physician* (London, 1724), pp. 181-2.
14 P Thickness, *A Letter to a Young Lady* (London, 1764), p. 11.
15 F Foster, *Thoughts for the Times but Chiefly on the Profligacy of Our Women* (London, 1779), pp. 6, 17-24, 31, 79.
16 For a more detailed account of these Charities and other voluntary organisations see Jean Donnison, *Midwives and Medical Men* (Heinneman, 1977), p. 27-8.
17 Quoted in *Nursing Times*, 4 January, 1947.
18 G Clark, *A History of the College of Physicians* (Oxford, 1964-72), Vol. II, p. 588.
19 Sir H Halford to Sir R Peel, March 1827, College of Physicians, *Annals*, 11 May 1827.
20 J M Munro Kerr (ed.), *Historical Review of British Obstetrics and Gynaecology 1800-1950* (1954), pp. 332-3.
21 Francis B Smith, *The People's Health*, 1830-1916 (New York: Holmes & Meier, 1979), p. 23.
22 Ibid., p. 24.
23 Census findings reported in C Booth's *Life and Labour* (London, 1896), Vol. VIII.
24 Captain Marryat, *A Diary in America* (London, 1839) quoted in Duncan Crow, *The Victorian Woman* (George Allen & Unwin, 1971), pp. 28-9.
25 Letter signed 'A', Examiner (June, 1827).
26 Donnison, op. cit., p. 62.
27 Registrar-General, *Annual Report for 1876*, p. 250.
28 Select Committee on Protection of Infant Life, *Evidence*, Q.Q. 57, 791-809, 3760-1.
29 *Obstetrical Journal of Great Britain and Ireland*, Vol. I, p. 690.
30 *Lancet*, 1879, I, pp. 746-7.

31 Departmental Committee on the Midwives Act 1902, pp. 1909 XXXIII, *Evidence*, Q.Q. 2602-6.

Midwifery in America

1 Richard and Dorothy Wertz, *Lying-in* (New York: The Free Press, a Division of Macmillan, Inc, 1977), p. 11.
2 Charles Everton Nash, *The History of Augusta, Including the Diary of Nun Maither Moore Balland 1785-182* (Augusta, 1904), pp. 229-464.
3 Wyndham B Blanton, *Medicine in Virginia in the Seventeenth Century* (1930; reprint New York: Arno Press, 1972), p. 164.
4 Kenneth A Lockridge, 'The Population of Denham, Massachusetts, 1636-1736', *Economic History Review*, 2nd Series, 19 (1966), p. 331.
5 Quoted in Adrienne Rich, *Of Woman Born* (Virago, 1977), p. 137.
6 For a fuller expansion on the theory of the elimination of magic and the position of the midwife see Wertz, op. cit., pp. 23-5.
7 Wertz, op. cit., p. 30.
8 Valentine Seaman, *The Midwive's Monitor and Mother's Mirror* (New York, 1800); Lewis Scheffey, 'The Early History and the Transitional Period of Obstetrics and Gynaecology in Philadelphia', *Annals of Medical History*, 3rd Series, 2 (May, 1940), pp. 215-24.
9 John B Blake, 'Woman and Medicine in Ante-Bellum America', *Bulletin of the History of Medicine*, 34, no. 2 (March-April, 1965), pp. 108-9; Dr Thomas Ewell, *Letters to Ladies* (Philadelphia, 1817), pp. 21-31.
10 *Buffalo Medical Journal*, 6 (Sept., 1850), pp. 250-1.
11 John Stearns, 'Presidential Address', *Transactions of the New York State Medical Society*, 1, p. 139.
12 Anonymous, *Remarks on the Employment of Females as Practitioners in Midwifery* (Boston, 1820).
13 Charles D Meigs, *Females and Their Diseases: A Series of Letters to His Class* (Philadelphia, 1848), pp. 41-2, 46-7.
14 Elizabeth Blackwell, 'Address on the Medical Education of Women', Dec. 27, 1855 (New York, 1856), pp. 4-6.

BIRTH — THE GROWTH OF THE MEDICAL APPROACH

1 Quoted in Brian Inglis, *A History of Medicine* (Weidenfeld & Nicolson), p. 49.
2 This title was given Harvey by J H Aveling a prominent nineteenth-century obstetrician and author of *English Midwives: Their History and Prospects*. See also Harvey Graham, Eternal Eve (Hutchinson, 1950), p. 136.
3 Quoted in Harvey Graham, op. cit., pp. 144-5.
4 P Willughby, *Observations in Midwifery*, H Blenkinsop (ed.) (Warwick, 1863), pp. 248-9.
5 Quoted in Harvey Graham, op. cit., p. 144.
6 Ibid., 156.

7 Ibid., 156.
8 Ibid., 165-6.
9 Ibid., 154.
10 Duncan Stewart, 'The Caesarean Operation Done with Success by a Midwife', in *Medical Essays and Observations*, 5 (1752), 360-2.
11 Charles White, *Treatise on the Management of Pregnancy and Lying-in Women, and the Means of Curing, but more especially of Preventing the Principal Disorders to which they are Liable* (1772), quoted in Graham, op. cit., pp. 195-6.
12 Lawrence Stone, *The Family, Sex and Marriage in England 1500-1800* (Weidenfeld & Nicolson, 1977), pp. 77-8.
13 Harvey Graham, op. cit., p. 233.
14 *New England Quarterly Journal of Medicine and Surgery*, April, 1843.
15 O Wendell Holmes, *Puerperal Fever a Private Pestilence* (Boston, 1855), p. 60.
16 Quoted in Graham, op. cit., p. 211.
17 Ibid., p. 215.
18 Ibid., p. 220.
19 Ibid., p. 220.
20 Myrtle Simpson, *Simpson the Obstetrician* (Victor Gollancz, 1972), p. 39.
21 From the *American Journal of Surgery: Anaesthesia Supplement* (1915), vol. 29, p. 101.
22 H L Gordon, *Sir James Young Simpson and Chloroform*, (1897) p. 106.
23 Fleetwood Churchill, *Theory and Practice of Midwifery* (1872) 6th edn, p. 341.
24 J M Munro Kerr (ed.), *Historical Review of British Obstetrics and Gynaecology 1800-1950* (1954), pp. 79-80.

THE TWENTIETH CENTURY

The early years

1 Margaret Llewelyn Davies, *Maternity: Letters from Working Women*, London 1978.
2 British Parliamentary Papers, 'Report of the Inter-Departmental Committee on Physical Deterioration,' vol 1, 1904, Cd 2175, XXXII, i.
3 Board of Education, Annual Report for 1914, London HMSO.
4 Jane Lewis, *The Politics of Motherhood*, London 1980, p. 16.
5 Annual Report of the Medical Officer of Health for St Pancras, 1090, p. 3, and Charles Porter, *The Future Citizen and His Mother*, Constable 1918, p. 11.
6 J W Ballantyne, *Manual of Ante-Natal Pathology and Hygiene*, Edinburgh 1904.
7 WCG, Memo on the National Care of Maternity, Guild 1917, p. 1.
8 J M Campbell, *Maternal Mortality*, Reports on Public Health and Medical Subjects, No 25, MOH, London 1924, p. 5.
9 S Pankhurst, *Save the Mothers*, London 1930, p. 46.

10 Ministry of Health, Final Report of the Committee on Maternal Mortality, HMSO 1932, p. 13.

11 PRO, MH55/679, Circular 1622, 7 May 1937.

12 Baird wrote: 'Like pioneers in other fields, Britain made many mistakes during her industrial development which those who industrialised later were able to avoid . . . as a result of those social and economic influences, many women in Britain suffered a considerable reduction in their reproductive efficiency, as measured by stillbirth and perinatal mortality rates, due to environmental conditions which they experienced when they were young children, or even *in utero*.' Sir Dugald Baird, BJO 87, no 12, Dec. 1980, p. 1058, 'Environment and Reproduction'.

13 Sir Dugald Baird, 'The Changing Pattern of Human Reproduction in Scotland, 1928-72', Fourth Marie Stopes Memorial Lecture, J Biosoc. Sci. (1975) 7, 77-97.

14 Mary Thomson, *Stork's Nest*, unpublished manuscript.

15 MOH (1927), *The Protection of Motherhood*, J M Campbell, Reports on Public Health and Medical Subjects No 25, London HMSO, p. 6.

16 Llewelyn Davies, op. cit., p. 16.

17 Departmental Committee on Maternal Mortality and Morbidity (1930) *Interim Report*, London HMSO, p. 39.

18 PRO, MH55/262, Newman to Secretary, 26 October 1932.

19 Peter Gabriele Filene, *Himf Herf Self: Sex Roles in Modern America*, New York 1975, p. 46.

20 S Josephine Baker, 'Why do Our Babies Die?', *Ladies Home Journal 40*, October 1923, pp. 212-13.

21 WCG, *Memo on the National Care of Maternity*, p. 4.

22 Llewelyn Davies, op. cit., p. 20.

23 Ibid, p. 22.

24 Robert Anderson, letter to the *BMJ*, 2 July 1921, p. 28.

25 Mary Thomson, *Stork's Nest*.

26 Ibid.

27 Llewelyn Davies op. cit., p. 32.

28 Flora Thomson, *Lark Rise to Candelford*, p. 138.

29 *BMJ*, 7 June 1952, p. 1246.

30 'Report on a National Maternity Service', RCOG, London 1944.

31 Mary Thomson, op. cit.

32 New York Academy of Medicine Committee on Public Health Relations, 'Maternal Mortality in New York City: A Study of All Puerperal Deaths, 1930-32', New York 1933, pp. 32, 49, 186.

33 White House Conference on Child Health and Protection, Fetal, Newborn, and Maternal Mortality and Morbidity, New York 1933, pp. 215-17.

34 Richard and Dorothy Wertz, *Lying-in*, New York 1977, p. 164.

35 Louis S Reed, 'Midwives, Chiropodists and Optometrists: Their Place in Medical Care', No 15, Chicago 1932, pp. 17-19.

36 Mary Thomson, op. cit.

37 Ann Oakley, *The Captured Womb, A History of the Medical Care of Pregnant Women*, Oxford 1984, p. 142.

38 Sir D Baird, 'The Evolution of Modern Obstetrics', *Lancet*, 10 September 1960, pp. 557-64.

39   Norman White, quoted in W R Merrington, *UCL and its Medical School: A History*, London 1976, pp. 148-9.
40   Interview with Sir Dugald Baird in 'Profile', BBC Radio Scotland, 1979.
41   Andrew Topping, 'Prevention of Maternal Mortality', *Lancet* 7 March 1936, p. 546.
42   Douglas Miller, 'Observations on Unsuccessful Forceps Cases', *BMJ* August 1928, p. 183.
43   W Japp Sinclair, 'The Injuries of Parturition: The Old and the New', *BMJ* 4 September 1897, p. 595.
44   Flora Thomson, op. cit. p. 141.
45   Parliamentary Papers, '79th Annual Report of the Registrar General for 1916', 1917-18, vi 1 p. xxxiv.
46   Henry Jellett, *Causes and Preventions of Maternal Mortality*, London 1929, p. 238.
47   Janet Campbell, Ministry of Health, Reports on Public Health, 'Maternal Mortality', No 25, London 1924, p. 56.
48   A MacGregor, *Public Health in Glasgow 1905-46*, Edinburgh 1967.
49   Oakley, op. cit., p. 119.
50   Cranbrook Committee (1959) *Report of the Maternity Services Committee*, London HMSO.
51   Letters to the *Ladies' Home Journal*, 1958.
52   Ibid.
53   Ibid.
54   Ibid.
55   Mary Thomson, op. cit.
56   Interview with Sir Dugald Baird, Edinburgh 1983.
57   Interview with Sir Dugald Baird for 'Profile', BBC Radio Scotland, 1979.
58   Grantly Dick Read, *Childbirth Without Fear*, London 1942, 9th ed., p. 29.
59   Labour Party, Report of the 34th Conference, 1934, p. 182.
60   *BMJ*, 24 April 1954.
61   Ministry of Health, *Report of the Maternity Services Committee*, 1959, (Cranbrook Report), HMSO, London.
62   DHSS, 'Domiciliary midwifery and maternity bed needs', HMSO, (Peel Report), London 1970.
63   Ibid.
64   Cranbrook Report, 1959.
65   Second Report from the Social Services Committee (the Short Report), *Perinatal and Neonatal Mortality*, HMSO London 1980.
66   Jane Lewis, *The Politics of Motherhood*, London 1980, p. 21.

Medical change

1   Sheila Kitzinger and John A Davies (eds.), *The Place of Birth*, Oxford 1978, p. 47.
2   H W Florey et al., *Lancet* 2, 177, 1941.

3   J Smith, 'Causation and Source of Infection in Puerperal Fever', Edinburgh 1931, HMSO; and Dora C Colebrook, 'The Source of Infection in Puerperal Fever due to Haemolytic Streptococci', Medical Research Council, Special Rep. Series, No 205, London 1936, HMSO.

4   Eliza Taylor Ransome Papers, Schlesinger Library, Radcliffe College, quoted in Wertz, *Lying-nn*, New York 1977.

5   Joseph B DeLee, 'The Prophylactic Forceps Operation', *AJO and G 1*, 1920, pp. 34-44.

6   J M Munro Kerr, James Hay Ferguson, James Young and James Henry, *A Combined Textbook of Obstetrics and Gynaecology*, Edinburgh 1923, p. 320.

7   Minutes of the Meeting of the Council of the Medical Women's Federation, vol II, 26 October 1928, MWF Archives.

8   James D Voorhees, 'Can the Frequency of some Obstetrical Operations be Diminished?' *AJO 77*, 1918, pp. 5, 9.

9   Albert H Aldridge and Richard S Meredith, 'Obstetric Responsibility for the Prevention of Foetal Deaths', *AJO and G 42*, 1941, p. 388.

10   Emanuel A Friedman, 'Graphic Analysis of Labour', *Bulletin of the American College of Nurse-Midwifery*, 1959, p. 97.

11   A MacFarlane, 'Variations in Number of Births and Perinatal Mortality by Day of the Week in England and Wales', *BMJ 2*, 1978, pp. 1670-3.

12   'A Time to be Born', *Lancet*, 1974, ii, p. 1183.

13   Danae Brook, *Naturebirth*, London 1976; quotation from *Lancet*, 16 November 1974, p. 1183.

14   Ricardo L Schwartz et. al., 'Fetal Monitoring in spontaneous labours and elective inductions', *AJO and G 120*, 1974, pp. 356-62.

15   *Lancet*, 16 November 1974.

16   Fielding Ould, *A Treatise of Midwifery*, Dublin 1742, pp. 145-6.

17   Norman R Kretzschmar, 'A Study of 2987 Consecutive Episiotomies', *AJO and G 35*, 1938, pp. 621-2.

18   Nicholas J Eastman, *Williams Obstetrics*, 10th ed., 1950, New York, p. 412.

19   Sheila Kitzinger, 'Some Women's Experiences of Episiotomy', National Childbirth Trust, London 1981.

20   Henry Jellett, *Causes and Prevention of Maternal Mortality*, London 1929, p. 220.

21   Sir Dugald Baird, 'The Evolution of Modern Obstetrics', *Lancet*, 10 September 1960.

22   Nancy Wainer Cohen and Lois J Estner, *Silent Knife: Caesarean Prevention and Vaginal Birth after Caesarean*, Massachusetts 1983.

The Tide Turns

1   Richard and Dorothy Wertz, *Lying-in*, New York 1977, p. 173.

2   Grantly Dick Read, *Childbirth Without Fear*, London 1942, 9th ed. p. ix.

3   Ibid., p. 9.

4   Ibid., p. 90.

5 Ibid., p. 96.
6 Ibid., p. 97.
7 Barbara Katz Rothman, *In Labour, Women and Power in the Birthplace*, London 1982, pp. 87-8.
8 Betty Friedan, *The Feminine Mystique*, New York, 1963.
9 Marjorie Karmel, *Thank You Dr Lamaze: A Mother's Experiences in Painless Childbirth*, Philadelphia, 1959.
10 Frederique Leboyer, *Birth Without Violence*, Fontana, London 1975, p. 8.
11 Ibid., p. 10.
12 Michel Odent, *Entering the World: The De-Medicalisation of Childbirth*, London 1984, p. 34.
13 Ibid, p. 113.
14 Judith Dickson Luce, 'Birth Without Mothers: More Violence Against Women', *Monthly Extract*, May§June 1976.
15 *In Labour*, p. 100.
16 Judith Luce, op. cit.
17 Michel Odent, op. cit., p. 99.
18 Michel Odent, *Genèse de l'Homme Ecologique: L'Instinct Retrouvé*, Paris 1979.
19 *Mothering*, Fall 1983, p. 61.
20 Ibid., p. 60.
21 Janet Isaacs Ashford (ed), *The Whole Birth Catalog*, New York 1983, p. 41.
22 Sheila Kitzinger, *Birth at Home*, Oxford 1979, p. 6.
23 Ibid., pp. 3-4.
24 Second Report from the Social Services Committee *Perinatal and Neonatal Mortality* (The Short Report), London 1980, HMSO.
25 Kitzinger and Davies (eds), op. cit., pp. 85-92.
26 Ibid, pp. 93-117.
27 Ibid., p. 115.
28 Ann Oakley, *The Captured Womb*, Oxford 1984, p. 240.
29 AIMS Newsletter, October 1978, p. 1.
30 AIMS objectives, 1981.
31 See, for example *The Sunday Times*, 13 October 1974, Oliver and Louise Gillie, 'The Childbirth Revolution'.
32 Leaflet issued by the Association of Radical Midwives, 'Discussion Points', by Thelma Bamfield.

The growth of antenatal care

1 J W Ballantyne, *Manual of Ante-Natal Pathology and Hygiene*, I The Foetus, Edinburgh 1902.
2 *BMJ* 6 April 1901.
3 J H Ferguson, 'Some Twentieth Century Problems in Relation to Marriage and Childbirth', Transactions of the Edinburgh Obstetrical Society, 1912, vol 38, pp. 3-39.
4 Ibid., p. 4.

5   W L MacKenzie, *Scottish Mothers and Children*, Dunfermline, 1917, p. 51.
6   'A National Maternity Service', *BMJ* Supplement, 29 June 1929, p. 260.
7   Mary Thomson, *Stork's Nest*.
8   Ibid.
9   Ibid.
10 Ann Oakley, *The Captured Womb*, Oxford 1985, p. 94.
11 Quoted in Jill Rakusen and Nick Davidson, *Out of Our Hands*, London 1982, p. 29.
12 *The House of Commons Social Services Committee on Perinatal and Neonatal Mortality* (The Short Report), House of Commons Paper 663§1, HMSO 1980.
13 Sir Dugald Baird, 'Environment and Reproduction', *BJO and G* vol 87 No 12, Dec 1980.
14 H Graham, 'Smoking in Pregnancy; the attitude of expectant mothers', *Social Science and Medicine*, vol 10, pp. 399-405, 1976.
15 M H Hall, P K Chng and I MacGillivray, 'Is routine antenatal care worthwhile?', *Lancet* 12 July 1980, p. 78.
16 Ibid.
17 *Lancet*, 15 March 1980.
18 *BMJ* 19 August 1980.
19 Hall, Chng and MacGillivray, op. cit.
20 Catherine Boyd and Lea Sellers (eds), *The British Way of Birth*, London 1982.
21 Ibid.
22 Ibid.
23 Ibid.
24 *British Births 1970*, London 1975.
25 Departmental Committee on Maternal Mortality and Morbidity, Memorandum: 'Ante-natal Clinics: Their Conduct and Scope', *MOH* 1929, reprinted Departmental Committee 1930.

FERTILITY AND CHOICE

The evolution of birth control

1   August Forel, *Sexual Ethics*, 1908, English translation, p. 62.
2   *Lancet, 1873*.
3   Carl Djerassi, *The Politics of Contraception, The Present and the Future*, San Francisco, 1979, p. xvii.
4   Genesis 38, v. 8-10.
5   Shirley Green, *The Curious History of Contraception*, London 1971, p. 30.
6   Germaine Greer, *Sex and Destiny, The Politics of Human Fertility*, London 1984, pp. 109-10.
7   Green, op. cit., p. 68.
8   *Tatler*, 1709, quoted Green, op. cit., p. 77.
9   James Boswell, *London Journal*, 25 March 1763.

10 Ibid., 4 June 1763.
11 Green, op. cit., p. 17.
12 *Le Rideau Leve*, 1786, quoted Green, op. cit., p. 102.
13 Marie Stopes, *Contraception, Theory, History and Practice*, 1941 ed., pp. 164-6.
14 H A Allbutt, *The Wife's Handbook*, London 1866.
15 Richard Carlile, *Every Woman's Book: or What is Love?*, London 1836.
16 Ibid.
17 Quoted in Stopes, op. cit., p. 305.
18 Carlile, op. cit., pp. 36-7.
19 Dr E Blackwell, 'How to Keep a Household in Health', London 1870, p. 8.
20 Green, op. cit., p. 73.
21 P Geddes and J A Thomson, *The Evolution of Sex*, London 1889.
22 Sidney Webb, *The Decline in the Birth Rate*, Italian Tract no. 131, London 1907.
23 Forel, op. cit.
24 Francis Galton, 'Eugenics, its definition, scope and aims', *Sociological Papers*, London 1905, p. 47.
25 Sir James Barr, President's Address to the 8th Annual Meeting of the BMA: 'What are we? What are we doing here? Whence do we come and whither do we go?' *BMJ* vol. ii, pp. 157-63, London, July 1912.
26 A Jacobi: President's Address before the American Medical Association at the 63rd session, Atlantic City, 'The Best Means of Combating Infant Mortality', *Journal of the Association*, vol. lviii, pp. 1737-44, Chicago, June 1912.
27 Marie Stopes, *Wise Parenthood, a sequel to Married Love: a book for Married People*, London 1918.
28 Stopes, *Contraception, Theory, History and Practice*, p. 327.
29 Marie Stopes, 'A Letter to Working Mothers on How to Have Healthy Children and Avoid Weakening Pregnancies', Leatherhead, 1919.
30 Margaret Lewelyn Davies, op. cit., p. 14.
31 *BMJ*, August 1921.
32 Professor Elaine M Wolfson, 'Effects of the Oral Contraceptive and its Meaning for Women', talk at the first Annual John Rock MD Commemorative Symposium, University of Pennsylvania School of Medicine, October 21, 1980.
33 Greer, op. cit., p. 134.
34 Ibid., p. 141.
35 Djerassi, op. cit.
36 Ibid., pxvii.
37 Ibid., p. 119.
38 Marge Berer, *Who needs Depo Provera*, London 1984.

Abortion – as old as life

1 Potts, Diggory and Peel, *Abortion*, Cambridge 1977, p. 2.
2 Carl Djerassi, *The Politics of Contraception, The Present and the Future*, San Francisco, 1979, p. 146.
3 ed Margaret Llewelyn Davies, *Maternity, Letters from Working Women*, reprinted London, 1978, pp. 24-5.
4 Avicenna, *Canon*.
5 trans. Beryl Rowland, *Mediaeval Woman's Guide to Health, the First Gynaecological Handbook*, London 1981, p. 121.
6 Ibid.
7 T Helie, 'De l'action veneneuse de la rue et de son influence sur la grossesse', *Annales d'hygiène et de médécine légales*, 20, 1838, pp. 181-2.
8 Jean Reneaux, 'A propos des propriétés abortives des essences de rue et de sabine, *Archives internationales de pharmacodynamie*, 66, 1941, p. 472.
9 van de Warkle, 'The detection of criminal abortion', *Journal of the Boston Obstetrical Society*, 5, 1870, p. 350.
10 Frederic Griffith, 'Instruments for the Production of Abortion sold in the Market Place of Paris', *Medical Record*, 30 January 1904, pp. 171-2.
11 Ibid.
12 Llewelyn Davies op. cit., p. xiii.
13 *BMJ* 1864, 2, p. 446.
14 Sir J Y Simpson, *Clinical Lectures on the Diseases of Women*, Edinburgh 1863.
15 Bernard M Dickens, *Abortion and the Law*, London 1966, p. 11.
16 Ibid., p. 13.
17 R R Rentoul, *The Causes and Treatment of Abortion, Edinburgh and London*, 1889.
18 *BMJ*, 1968.
19 D Reese, *Report on Infant Mortality in Large Cities*, 1910.
20 van de Warkel, op. cit., 4, 1870, p. 292.
21 E Shorter, *A History of Women's Bodies*, Toronto 1983, p. 223.
22 Sir Dugald Baird, 'A Fifth Freedom' *BMJ* 8, 13 Nov. 1965.
23 Dickens, op. cit., p. 121.
24 quoted in Potts et. al., op. cit., p. 285.
25 *Daily Telegraph*, 16 March 1965.
26 *The Times*, June 1965.
27 Potts et. al., op. cit., p. 308.
28 G E Godber, 'Abortion Deaths', *BMJ* 3, 1972, p. 424.
29 Report of the Committee on the working of the Abortion Act (1974), chairman the Hon: Mrs Justice Lane: vol 1 *Report*, vol ii *Statistical Volume*, HMSO, London. For a full account of the 1967 Abortion Act, its applications and implications, see Potts et. al. op. cit., pp. 277-330. Also Madeleine Simms and Keith Hindall, *Abortion Law Reformed*, London 1975.
30 Jean Smith, *The Scotsman*, January 26, 1984.
31 Potts et. al., op. cit., p. 411 (fig. 45).
32 Ibid., p. 2.

Infertility – a new technology

1 Robert Edwards and Patrick Steptoe, *A Matter of Life*, London 1980, p. 12.
2 Germaine Greer, *Sex and Destiny*, London 1984, p. 74.
3 Edwards and Steptoe, op. cit., p. 181.
4 Greer, op. cit. p. 49.
5 G Bettendorf, *Infertility: Diagnosis and Treatment of Functional Infertility*, Berlin 1978, p. ix.
6 Carl J Paverstein and Carlton A Eddy, 'The role of the oviduct in reproduction: our knowledge and our ignorance', Journal of Reproduction and Fertility, 55, pp. 223-9.
7 Greer, op. cit., p. 74.
8 Edwards and Steptoe, op. cit., p. 45.
9 Ibid., p. 106.
10 Ibid., p. 118.
11 Ibid., p. 109.
12 eds. William Walters and Peter Singer, *Test Tube Babies*, Oxford, 1982, p. 24.
13 Ibid., p. 34.
14 Edwards and Steptoe, op. cit., p. 96.
15 eds. Walters and Singer, op. cit., p. 84.
16 Report of the Committee of Inquiry into Human Fertilisation and Embryology, London HMSO 1984, Introduction.
17 Hansard, 15 February 1985, speech by Rt. Hon. Enoch Powell, M.P.
18 eds. Walters and Singer, op. cit., pp. 125, 126.

REVALUATIONS

1 Norman Morris, 'Human Relations in Obstetrics', *Lancet*, 23 April 1961, p. 915.
2 F W Smith, et. al., 'NMR Imaging in Human Pregnancy: A Preliminary Study', *Magnetic Resonance Imaging* vol 2, 1984, pp. 57-64.
3 Michel Odent, *Entering the World, The De- Medicalization of Childbirth*, New York and London 1984, p. 86.
4 *Mothering*, Fall 1983, p. 59.
5 Birth Centre London Leaflet, 'Episiotomy'.
6 Polly Toynbee, 'Natural Childbirth, a New Tyranny?', *Vogue*, May 1985.
7 RCOG report 1982, p. 27.
8 Odent, op. cit., p. 30.
9 Ivan Illich, *Medical Nemesis*, London 1975.
10 Sheila Kitzinger and John Davies (eds), *The Place of Birth*, Oxford 1978, p. 52.

Further Reading

Arms, S., *Immaculate Deception: A New Look at Women and Childbirth in America*, Boston 1975.

Berer, M., *Who Needs Depo Provera?* London 1984.

Betman, O., *A Pictorial History of Medicine*, Illinois, 1956.

Boyd, C. and Sellers, L. (eds), *The British Way of Birth*, London 1982.

Branca, P., *The Silent Sisterhood*, London 1975.

Branca, P., *Women in Europe since 1750*, London 1978.

Brook, D., *Naturebirth*, London 1976.

Cianfrani, T., *A Short History of Obstetrics and Gynaecology*, Illinois 1960.

Cutter, F. and Weits, S., *A Short History of Midwifery*, London 1964.

Davies, M. Llewelyn, *Maternity: Letters from Working Women*, London 1978.

Dickens, B. M., *Abortion and the Law*, London 1966.

Djerassi, C., *The Politics of Contraception, The Present and the Future*, San Francisco 1979.

Donnison, J., *Midwives and Medical Men*, London 1977.

Dow, D., *The Rottenrow: The History of the Glasgow Royal Maternity Hospital 1834-1984*, Glasgow 1984.

Edwards, R. and Steptoe, P., *A Matter of Life*, London 1980.

Ehrenreich, B. and English D., *Witches, Midwives and Women, A History of Women Healers*, London 1973.

Finney, R. P., *The Story of Motherhood*, New York 1937.

Fraser, A., *The Weaker Vessel*, London 1984.

Fried, P., *Pregnancy and Life Style Habits*, New York and Toronto 1983.

Friedan, B., *The Feminine Mystique*, New York 1963.

Graham, H., *Eternal Eve*, London 1960.

Green, S., *The Curious History of Contraception*, London 1971.

Greer, G., *Sex and Destiny, The Politics of Human Fertility*, London 1984.

Guthrie, D., *A History of Medicine*, London 1945.

Illich, I., *Medical Nemesis*, London 1975.

Inglis, B., *A History of Medicine*, London 1965.

Isaacs, J. Ashford, *The Whole Birth Catalog*, New York 1983.

Karmel, M., *Thank You Dr Lamaze: A Mother's Experiences in Painless Childbirth*, Philadelphia 1959.

Katz Rothman, B., *In Labour, Women and Power in the Birthplace*, London 1982.

Kitzinger, S. and Davies, J. A. (eds), *The Place of Birth*, Oxford 1978.

Kitzinger, S., *Birth at Home*, Oxford 1979.

Kitzinger, S., *The Experience of Childbirth*, London 1982.

Knibielher, Y. and Fouquet, C., *Histoire des mères du Moyen Age à nos jours*, Paris 1977.

Leboyer, F., *Birth Without Violence*, London 1975.

Lewis, J., *The Politics of Motherhood*, London 1980.

Marshall, R., *Virgins and Viragoes*, London 1983.

Munro Kerr, J. M. (ed), *Historical Review of British Obstetrics and Gynaecology 1800-1950*, Edinburgh 1954.

Oakley, A., *The Captured Womb*, Oxford 1984.

Odent, M., *Entering the World: The De-Medicalization of Childbirth*, London 1984.

Pankhurst, S., *Save the Mothers*, London 1930.

Potts, Diggory and Peel, *Abortion*, Cambridge 1977.

Radcliffe, W., *Milestones of Midwifery*, Bristol 1967.

Rakusen, J. and Davidson, N., *Out of Our Hands*, London 1982.

Read, D. Grantly, *Childbirth Without Fear*, London 1942.

Rich, A., *Of Woman Born*, London 1977.

Riley, M., *Brought to Bed*, London 1968.

Rowland, B., *Medieval Woman's Guide to Health*, Ohio 1981.

Shorter, E., *A History of Women's Bodies*, New York 1982.

Simms, M. and Hindall, K., *Abortion Law Reformed*, London 1975.

Simpson, M., *Simpson the Obstetrician*, London 1972.

Stone, L., *The Family, Sex and Marriage in England 1500-1800*, London 1977.

Stopes, M., *Contraception, History, Theory and Practice*, London 1941.

Stopes, M., *Wise Parenthood, a sequel to Married Love: a book for Married People*, London 1918.

Wainer Cohen, N. and Estner, L. J., *Silent Knife: Caesarean Prevention and Vaginal Birth after Caesarean*, Massachusetts 1983.

Wertz, R. and D., *Lying In*, New York 1977.

Zander, L. and Chamberlain, G., *Pregnancy Care for the 1980s*, London 1984.

List of Abbreviations

AJO American Journal of Obstetrics
AJO & J American Journal of Obstetrics and Gynaecology
BJO British Journal of Obstetrics
BMA British Medical Association
BMJ British Medical Journal
BJO British Journal of Obstetrics
HMSO Her Majesty's Stationery Office
MOH Ministry of Health
NHS National Health Service
PRO Public Records Office
WCG Women's Co-operative Guild

INDEX

abortifacient poisons, 226-7
abortion, 11, 133, 201, 202, 218, 222-236, *235*
Abortion Act, 234-5
Abortion Law Reform Association (ALRA), 233, *233*
Accouchement Forcé, 118
Active Birth Movement, 186
AIMS, 186
Allbutt, Arthur, 213-14
alphafetaprotein, *191*, 192, 195, 247
Ambrose, 15
American Birth Control League, 217
American Board of Obstetrics and Gynaecology, 145
American Gynaecological Society, 172
American Medical Association, 89, 138, 215
American Society for Psychoprophylaxis in Obstetrics (ASPO), 179
amniocentesis, 191, 247
anaesthesia, 51-4, *52*, 112, *117*, 118-20, 139, 140, 155, 162, 167-70, 174, 176, 177, 178, 228, 229
analgesia, 139, 140, 149, 155, 156, 167-71, 172, 177, 183
Anderson, Elizabeth Garrett, 81, 82-3
antenatal care, 132, 158, 185, 187-98, *189*, *191*, *192*, *193*
anthrax, 122
antibiotics, 10, 146, 164, *165*, 166
antisepsis, 44, 54, 55, *117*, 123
Apergol, 228
apiol, 227-8
Apothecaries, Society of, 76, 81, 83
Aristotle, 18
Ascheim-Zondek, 247
asepsis, 119, 120, 123, 140, 144, 146, 171, 177
Association of Radical Midwives, 186
Augustin, 15
Avicenna, 223

Jacobs, Alletta, 213
Jacquemier, J M, 49
Jellett, Henry, 154
Jenner, Edward, 109
Jerome, 15
Joceline, Elizabeth, 31
Jones, Margaret, 86
Joret, 227

Karman, Harvey, 228
Karmel, Marjorie, 179
Karmin, 229
Kehrer, F A, 119
Kitzinger, Sheila, 184
Knowlton, Charles, 207, 211
Koch, Robert, 122, 124, 162

Ladies Home Journal, 138, 155
Ladies Medical College, 81
Lamaze, Ferdinand, 179
Lancet, 173
Landsteiner, Karl, 122, 166
Lane Committee, 234
Lang, Raven, 183
laparoscope, 240
Lathrop, Julia, 137, 138
Lawson Tait, Robert, 119
Leboyer, Frederique, 179-82, 183
Leeuwenhoek, Anthony van, 122
Levret, Andre, 104
Lewis, Jane, 161-2
Lister, Joseph, *117*, 121, 123
Liston Robert, 117, *117*
lithotomy *see* birthing positions
Local Government Act, 14
London Blood Transfusion Service, 166
London School of Medicine for Women, 83
Long, Crawford, 118
Louis XIV, 71
lying-in, 29-30, 142, 185
lying-in hospitals, 43-4, 75, 80, 104, 114, 115, 173, 187, 188

McDowell, Ephraim, 110, *111*
malpresentation, 34-5, 37, 60
Malthusian League, 213, 214
Malthusian Quackery, 212
Manningham, Sir Richard, 74-5, 102
Married Love, 215